Zaïda

There is only one requirement
for a woman to be able to belly dance...
she must be able to have FUN

Zaïda

Belly Dancing for Older Women

Zaïda

Writers Club Press
San Jose New York Lincoln Shanghai

Writers Club Press
an imprint of iUniverse, Inc.

For information address:
iUniverse, Inc.
5220 S. 16th St., Suite 200
Lincoln, NE 68512
www.iuniverse.com

ISBN: 0-595-20948-3

Printed in the United States of America

Zaïda

Bellydancing for Older Women

I dedicate this book to my husband, Mike.

Mike has supported me every step of the way
in my quest to learn belly dancing
and to educate the uninitiated in the sheer joy,
and the physical and mental benefits
of this dance.

I thank also, my long suffering, but meticulous Proof Readers.

Author: Zaïda

Index

website *http://welcome.to/Zaida*

CHAPTER 1

Zaïda

website: http://welcome.to/Zaida

Belly Dancing for Older Women

Zaïda means 'lucky'.

'Belly Dancing' evokes visions of harem girls dancing in very skimpy costumes for the entertainment and titillation of the Sheik. The fabled *'Dance of the Seven Veils'* always springs from the lips of the uninitiated.

This is pure Hollywood hype. Oscar Wilde is reputed to have evoked the *Dance of the Seven Veils* from his fantasies. The Western image of harems stems from the Victorian era when anything vaguely sexual was highly prized on the black-market, due to the extreme repressions of the era. Authors wrote their wildest fantasies as factual reports of life in the harem. Not one of them would have gained access to a harem or lived to tell the tale had they done so.

Everything the Western world thinks it knows about harems is pure fantasy

Belly Dancing—Baladi (pronounced Beh-leh-dee and mistaken for Belly), is a health regimen which has evolved over the centuries. The origins of the dance are extremely ancient, predating Islam, Christianity and

3

even Judaism. The dance has no affiliation with current religion anywhere in the world.

It encompasses all the aspects of the human entity. The physical, psychological, emotional, social and financial aspects of that entity.

In the West, the dance has evolved by absorbing the 'best' from the dances of many countries, not only the Middle East, and is thus an amorphous blending of many styles.

PHYSICAL—You will gain enormous strength, vitality and flexibility. This does not mean you will become muscle-bound and masculine looking. It means that your muscles will regain the flexibility of youth. You will be able to move more freely and will particularly notice this new-found strength when descending stairs; you will not need to cling to the railings.

Your balance will improve and you will be unlikely to fall, even on difficult ground. One of the greatest fears of older women is to break a hip, as this will affect them for the rest of their lives and possibly mean they will need a walking stick to aid with mobility.

Muscle strength also means excellent weight control as muscle burns fat, so, although your weight may not change much, your body will become trim and finely defined as you rebuild your muscles. You will be able to consume larger quantities of food without depositing fatty layers. As muscle is heavier than fat, your scales will not give you much reassurance, so ignore the scales and just concentrate on how you 'feel' and look.

Best of all, you will feel enormously energetic and vibrant. You will feel STRONG.

PSYCHOLOGICAL—You will experience a deep-seated sense of self-worth. You will feel totally self-possessed and in control of your life. You will know who you are and that you are a very worthwhile person.

You may not be the 'BEST' dancer in the world, but you will be unique. You will be YOU. Nobody can possibly bring to the dance just what you can bring. Whether it be verve and vivacity, delicate shades of meaning, comedy or pathos; you will interpret the dance according to your personality and you will find your dance changing as your psyche blossoms.

You will feel sure of yourself as a woman. Your walk will show the world how you feel about yourself. You will glow with good health. You will be FIT.

EMOTIONAL—Many women find it difficult or even impossible to express their emotions. Their past experiences may have frozen them into a protective shell in order that they may not be hurt, ridiculed or exploited.

Their upbringing may have left them with a major overburden of inhibitions. One dancer could not move her upper body, no matter how hard she tried. She was big busted and had been told all her formative years, not to flaunt herself, so she had learned to keep her chest area very understated; hidden under loose clothing and never, ever displayed.

Other dancers would KILL for such charms.

Another dancer could not move her hip section. She would try and try but it was absolutely frozen. She never divulged the reason for her frozen pelvis. She never spoke about her private life or her childhood.

We, in the class, threatened to join the two together by taking the top of one and the bottom of the other, to make one flexible dancer......

Both these dancers eventually started to loosen up and as they continued with their dancing, they gradually overcame their brain-washed mind-set.

Their personalities blossomed.

The dance will release all these pent-up emotions and a new dancer may even find herself sobbing as she dances. These negative emotions will pass and the sheer joy of the dance will shine through. Whenever a dancer hears music with a driving beat, and it need not be Arabic music, she will find herself responding to that music with an almost irresistible urge to dance.

Best of all…. if she does get up to dance, she will be able to surprise everyone present with her grace and ability.

SOCIAL—You will have a *party piece* to entertain your friends. How many times have you enjoyed someone else doing something entertaining at a social function and wishing you could do 'something'? Well, belly dancing will knock their eyes out. Many of them will be envious, lets face it, downright jealous, not only of your ability to do the moves, but your self-confidence in being able to entertain.

You will gain a whole new circle of friends and if you are on the Internet you will find you are part of a worldwide sub-culture. Your interest in belly dancing will open doors you never even knew existed and you will learn about the day-to-day lives of people from the most exotic places. This is far more interesting than doing the tourist thing and seeing only the 'beautiful scenery'.

FINANCIAL—This is reflected in the coins and golden jewellery worn by belly dancers. Originally this represented a woman's entire wealth and was worn in order to keep it safe. In the West, it is purely decorative.

Many dancers make an extremely good living out of their dancing, indeed, the most famous belly dancers in Egypt are amongst the wealthiest women, in their own right; but this is not the prime focus—even these dancers would find their lives totally empty if they retired and did not dance.

Of course, none of this comes cheaply. You will have to work at your dancing and your attitude to life. You will discover that fellow dancers, throughout the world, will support you, encourage you and wish you well.

AUTHENTIC is just another hype word. This word has lost its true meaning, as has the word 'unique'. There is nothing authentic about 'belly dance'. This is the dance of the people and evolves and mutates as people move around the world and see new moves, which they include in their dance. It has always been thus, even in the early days of nomads and camel caravans. The Gypsies travelled around and spread their style of dance throughout the Middle East. As they discovered new styles and moves, they included these in their dances and took these moves to other places.

Belly dance is a 'living' dance; just as English is a 'living' language. Latin died because it was a rigid language and could not evolve with the needs of the people. English has survived and grown because it has adopted all the words from other languages which express a precise meaning; particularly in this technological age.

Thus belly dancers are constantly adopting ideas from different cultures and even from individual dancers. What goes around, comes around. This is what makes belly dancing so vital and vibrant.... it is expressing the feelings of the people NOW.

"We need to redefine age. Anything up to 60 is young.
60 to 80 is middle age and over 90 is elderly".

Ita Buttrose.

CHAPTER 2

CREATING YOUR COSTUME

&

CHOOSING COLOURS

There is no 'uniform' costume for Belly Dancing—in Australia; or possibly anywhere else. Follow your own inclination. You understand your figure perfections and imperfections better than anyone.

It is essential to dress in context in order to gain the true feel of the dance. You cannot see what a shimmy does when you are wearing bicycle shorts.... nothing moves. A figure eight and a circle don't become visible until something moves in the pattern. A rib shift under a loose tee shirt is completely invisible. You will feel you are not able to learn this dance.

I have found that new dancers are too embarrassed to hang their skirts from their hips. They are terrified that the skirt will 'fall off', or, they dislike the feel of the weight hanging from their hips. For those dancers who lack confidence in skirts hanging from their hips, they could wear very tight fitting bikini swimsuit bottoms, and safety pin the skirt to the bikini as added security. For myself, I thread very heavy, wide elastic through the waistline. I make sure it has reached the absolute limit of its stretch when

11

it fits tightly around my hips, thus there is no more stretch left to allow it to slide over my hip bones.

One dancer, who is very heavy in the thighs, made lightweight harem pants in a contrasting colour, and over this wore a Turkish skirt, the kind with a narrow front panel and the rest of the skirt flows around the back, forming two front slits from hem to the waist equidistant from the centre line. That is, the front panel is narrow and the rest of the skirt is not joined to the front panel and forms a three quarter circle from the front panel around the back to the front panel again. The effect is very slimming.

Pinning the skirt, or using a knotted hip scarf, a tightly knotted tassel belt or a metal link belt will also prevent the skirt falling off, no matter how vigorous the shimmy.

Hanging your skirt from your WAIST, defeats the whole purpose of the dance….which is to attract attention to the HIP movements. Until you hang your skirt from your hips, you will never experience the TRUE feel of the dance.

My preferred practice costume is a circle skirt hanging from hip level, joined to a top cut on princess lines and cut from stretch fabric with the s t r e t c h going sideways, so you do not need a zip. This dress is comfortable, flows beautifully, is easy to launder after class, and makes you FEEL like a dancer. You can see all the hip, waist, rib and shoulder movements.

Arm movements are enhanced by wearing sleeves or gauntlets, and these also hide bulges and sags.

The hip belt, which is essential, shows the shimmies and figure eights, so you can see you are making progress.

Many older women have beautiful legs and delicate ankles—design your costume to display this perfection in you. You may, in the beginning, have a thickened torso. Don't worry, this will soon diminish, much to your joy. In the meantime, design your costume to minimise the torso. This can be achieved in many ways with soft draping or decorative beads and fringes.

Experiment.

Costumes need not be expensive. You can raid the 'op' shops and buy pre-loved ball gowns and chop them up to your heart's content. You may even combine two or more gowns to achieve the effect you wish. In these shops you may even find beading or fringing attached to garments. Salvage the decorations and discard the garment.

Christmas decorations are usually very pretty and some are strong enough to withstand the demands of dancing. You would be amazed at how much punishment those strings of gold, silver or red beads can survive.

Plan your first costume just for classes. This way you will learn what adjustments you need to make in order to have a serviceable but comfortable costume. Also, your dancing in class will be enhanced when you are dressed in context. You will slip easily into your dancing persona. Leave your everyday self at the door. Enjoy yourself.

I made myself a costume out of a gold, knit fabric, which seemed so fragile it was likely to last only one wearing. This costume has absolutely astounded me by going on and on and on, without any signs of deterioration and surviving several bouts with the washing machine. It is beautiful to dance in as it flows and swirls and looks like liquid gold. The only thing it cannot tolerate is heat, so it cannot be ironed (does not need ironing) and I avoid sitting on the skirt—just in case.

One dancer bought a costume in Egypt. It was promised overnight and was duly delivered and looked absolutely beautiful, but when she got home and finally wore the costume in a performance (without looking too closely at the construction), she found it had been just loosely tacked together and even stapled in some places, and the bra almost fell off during her dance. Luckily she caught it in time and danced off stage, without the audience realising what had happened. She told me later, that she had to re-sew ALL the seams in the costume.

I find it is not necessary to finish off a costume too meticulously.... nobody is going to see it that closely. I never hem the bottom of the skirts, if the material does not fray, as this allows the skirt to flow much more freely. I just cut the hem with pinking shears and that suffices.

Sleeves do not need to be joined all around the armhole.... indeed, they allow more freedom of movement if they are only attached at the top of the shoulder; cooler too, as this style allows body heat to escape—and you get very HOT, dancing.

Avoid stays in the bodice of your dress. One dancer had a strapless dress, held up by stays, so of course, this made her ribcage rigid and she found her movements very limited. She looked terrific but the dress was totally useless for belly dancing.

Avoid materials which will create static electricity and cling to your legs. It may look 'sexy' but it will hinder your movements.

One dancer bought a very expensive beledi dress, which was liberally covered in *'Paillettes'*. Looked fantastic and flashed like gold lightning, but the paillettes kept catching on each other and causing the dress to strangle her legs.

My personal preference for a hardwearing, easily laundered skirt, is satin-backed crepe. Make the skirt with the shiny side out. This is a heavy material, it swirls beautifully and you don't have to bother too much about it whilst you are wearing it. You can sit down without creating any traumas and it is not a hot material to wear, as it is heavy enough to hang away from your body.

I like to wear a yashmak—my yashmak is a fine, gold chain, sari belt (Indian jewellery). It is pretty, hides the wrinkles, yet allows me to breathe.

People have said to me, *"I didn't know it was YOU"*.

My 45 year old son had several of my dancing photographs, which I had just emailed him, on display on his computer terminal.

His boss walked past and said, *'Is that work?'*.

My son said, *'No. That is my mother!'*.

'YEAH! RIGHT!', said his boss, totally disbelieving.

My husband, Mike, was talking with a lady who had been at a function where I had danced. She commented on the *'…really good belly dancer'*, she had seen.

Mike said to her, *'That is my wife'*.

'In your dreams', she retorted.

ILLUSION is the essence.

CHOOSING COLOURS

This item contributed by
Patricia Corbell, BSN, MA
Bachelor of Science in Nursing
Master of Arts, Philosophy and Religion
* (American spelling)

THE INFLUENCE OF COLOR

Color has a tremendous effect on all living beings.

White light from the sun is divided into a spectrum of colors which influence all areas of our lives.

Since ancient times, it has been known that colors influence our state of mind, our mood and even our personality. Students of color know that everyone needs exposure to each color in the spectrum to experience optimum health.

From early childhood, we develop preferences for certain colors and dislikes for others. Color psychology tests reveal that color preferences can be associated with personality types.

RED is the color of energy, vibrancy and action. A person who loves RED, may lean towards leadership, may enjoy physical activity and may take excessive risks.

ORANGE is the color of optimism, self-confidence and joy. One who favors ORANGE tends to have good self-esteem and loves being around people.

YELLOW is the color of optimism and happiness. It is associated with the mind, and one who loves YELLOW tends to be innovative and to accept different points of view.

GREEN is the color of healing and of harmony with nature. It is a calming, peaceful color and those who love GREEN tend to be conservative in their views.

BLUE is a cool, calming color and is associated with one's higher aspirations, as when one looks at the sky. One who favors BLUE tends to be idealistic and spiritual.

PURPLE is the color of intuition, creativity and mysticism. PURPLE transmutes impurities from the body and mind. Those who favor PURPLE may be reserved, artistic and dramatic.

PINK is the color of unconditional love. It is emotionally calming and those who love PINK may be considered nurturers.

As human beings, color influences every area of our lives from the physical body to the spirit. Those who study color can enhance their lives greatly and can improve their health and spiritual awareness.

The knowledge is there for the taking. I invite you to look more deeply into this exciting field.

'My sincere thanks to Patricia for her gift of time and information'.

Zaïda

ILLUSION AND ATMOSPHERE are the essence.

A three year old girl spoke to me
as I was loading my costume into my car, after a performance.
"Is that your's? It's pretty!", she said.
"Sure is", I replied, meaning it was mine and also that it was pretty.
"Why did you let the lady wear it?", she asked.
Made my day. She obviously did not realise that I was 'the lady'.

ILLUSION is the essence.

CHAPTER 3

ATTITUDE

*'Don't wait for the light at the end of the tunnel.
Stride down there and light the thing yourself.'*

The most difficult lesson for older women to learn—is how to overcome their upbringing—the rules which were drilled into their minds from infancy:

'Do not wiggle your hips'; 'Do not flaunt your bosom' (once you started to develop); Don't show off'; 'Don't draw attention to yourself'; 'Sit with your knees closed'; and the most often repeated instruction—

"If you act like a lady, you will be treated like a lady".

To ENJOY bellydancing, you must unlearn all these Do Not instructions—except the last one; that one still holds true in any situation. Always act like a lady.

You will find that as you progress into the intricacies of the dance, you will understand that you are NOT flaunting your body—you are expressing your inner self. The self you have always been instructed to suppress.

You will find a newborn sense of 'me'. You will be thrilled to experience your femininity. You will learn to "FLY" and release your soul. You will learn to be WOMAN.

When first experiencing bellydancing, many older women find that they cannot make LARGE movements with their arms. Their torsos are rigid and unyielding and they cannot raise their eyes to look at anyone else in the class.

Try to allow yourself six months trial, before deciding that bellydancing is not for you. You will never look back. Your friends will see a new person. Your husband will discover he has a new and exciting wife. You will feel much more calm and 'laid back' and let minor hassles just wash over you.

Once you are more relaxed with yourself and can accept that your body movements are an expression of the music, you will find a whole new world, which you did not know existed. Think of yourself as the music. Think of yourself as a musical note dancing to the tune. Think of yourself as anything other than an 'older woman'. You could have at least 30 years of dancing ahead of you. Enjoy yourself.

Discarding your inhibitions will improve the intimate areas of your life. Older women, having matured prior to the release of the Contraceptive Pill, grew up knowing that the only reliable form of contraception was the word 'NO'. When you mature with a specific mind-set, that will remain with you all your life, unless you deliberately work at changing your attitude. Bellydancing will free your mind as well as your body.

Do not try to get into other people's heads (especially your adult children); or worry about what they are thinking. They have to live their own lives. You have to live yours. You have no need to worry, or care, about what people think about your dancing.

The **nice people** will be happy for you, when they see how much you are enjoying yourself.

The others don't exist.

This is your play time. You have earned this time for yourself.

A very important aspect of taking charge of your **Attitude**, is that it directly affects your health. Scientific research has proven that people with a negative attitude are far more likely to have a weak immune system, thus laying themselves open to any infection or bacteria which happens their way.

'What you thought yesterday, you are living today; what you think today, you will live tomorrow'

The mind has enormous control over the processes of the human body; far more than has been proven with current knowledge. For instance, it was only in the last century that it was possible to examine a **living** brain. Now, scientists can see what parts of the brain are reacting to different stimuli and have even proven that male and female brains work differently (we all knew that anyway); the male brain focuses on one thought or activity at a time—hunting required total focus. The female brain is adapted to focus on many different thoughts and activities simultaneously—nurturing and caring and protecting the home. So, whereas the dead brains, when examined, appeared identical—the living brains are vastly different.

People with negative, despondent attitudes to life—expecting the worst, feeling they are not good enough, being sure they are going to 'catch' any illness going, responding especially to the media hypes.... well, they **will.**

People with positive attitudes to life—being sure their bodies are fit and well and perfectly capable of doing the job they are intended to do.... repel all boarders.... they will remain well. Their immune systems are functioning at optimum level.

Take note of all the people you know and you will see that the negative people are the ones who are always ill.

Think POSITIVE. Your body is designed to cope with bacteria and other forms of potential intruders. Maximise your body's fitness and you maximise your defences. Your mind is your most powerful defence; and the power of the mind is not yet fully understood....in Western society.

Learning to Teach

This is a major learning curve. You are dealing with a whole group of egos and personalities, not least of which are your own. You need to be able to lead these budding dancers into the light.... to let them understand that the dance is THEIR dance and not just a matter of ape-ing the teacher....*monkey see, monkey do.*

The dancers have to learn to LISTEN to the music and let their bodies flow and react to their feelings. This is very difficult for them as they may have never danced before. To move your body beyond the accustomed, socially prescribed movements, takes practice and determination. You have to learn to ignore your concerns that people may be critical or laughing at your efforts or even sneering. You don't need to live in their tiny minds. You need to live in your own mind, and when you feel the sheer JOY of dance you can be sure the tiny-minded people will never experience what you are experiencing at that moment.

To teach new dancers to move their bodies, you need to get them to start SMALL. Then slowly the movements will get bigger and bigger as they feel more comfortable about 'waving their arms around'. Hip movements are very difficult for new, older dancers, as they have held that part of their bodies RIGID for decades. We did not have the modern form of dance, where anything goes. We danced very sedate, social dances and the Jitterbug, which the American servicemen introduced us to, during the Second World War, was absolutely SHOCKING!

But exciting!

Chest movements are also a major problem for older dancers and they have to work slowly into the mind-set of actually moving that part of their body which they have always been told to minimise. Whenever I suggest to them that they imagine they have a tassel attached to each 'point' and try to swing them around, there is always great slightly embarrassed hilarity in the group. They are trying. Takes time. The important thing for the teacher, is to show them that it is not a matter for embarrassment, but a major health benefit, to MOVE that rib cage and thus massage all the internal organs in that part of the body. One learner stated that she felt 'silly and embarrassed' when she tried to move her 'chest' in front of an audience. She was happy to do the rib circles and lifts and drops, in class, but as soon as there was an audience her feelings changed. I explained, yet again, that Western women have great difficulty with these movements because of their childhood brainwashing. They just have to keep working at it as it is very important to move those ribs and massage those organs.

Little cheeky eye flicks at the audience are also something which has to be taught. I instil in my dancers that they should aim at pleasing individuals in the audience without causing them embarrassment; so I urge them to only look at a particular individual once, or at most twice....

unless he is absolutely captivating and you *'can't take my eyes off of you'....*

Smiles are spontaneous and not fixed grimaces. I would rather the dancers did not smile at all if they have to force a smile. They will find they cannot help, but smile, when they really start to DANCE.

When dancers start to HEAR and FEEL the music.... they will experience the sheer JOY of dancing. To become aware of the moment when a dancer suddenly hears the music.... that is a moment of delight, for the teacher.

In the Arabic countries, Baladi is learned from infancy, so the children learn to interpret the music according to their own feelings. This is what Western dancers have to learn as adults.

I had been asked by a number of women, over a period of at least three years, whether I taught belly dancing, and I kept saying, *"No! I don't teach!"* I held this attitude because I have never, ever enjoyed teaching anyone, anything. Particularly when I was handing over my job to the next incumbent. The process irritated me intensely; but teaching a group of very interested and eager dancers is pure pleasure. I am truly enjoying teaching in this situation.

I have found that it is best to teach new dancers one or two simple, structured dances, so they learn to move as a cohesive group, then to teach them two un-structured dances where they have to listen to the music and feel the moves which the music creates for them.

They tend to feel they are very scrappy and just flitting around, but I tell them that it is all movement and colour and they look absolutely beautiful when I look at them without my glasses (I always dance without my glasses).... this raises a good laugh and stops them feeling so intense.

I have also found that new dancers sometimes have great difficulty with the simplest movements but 'catch on' to trickier movements within a couple of attempts. Also 'left' and 'right' cause major traumas. I use several kinesiology movements in my warm-up, as this teaches the right side of the brain (artistic) to talk to the left side of the brain (logic). Many of these movements are derived from Yoga, Tai Chi or Brain Gym.

Most of the first students to join my class, had names beginning with 'J', so I have named my troupe *Zaïda's Jacarandas*. At our first public performance, at a Nursing Home, I asked the 'spare' dancers to stand in the background, during a duet performance, making sure they did not obscure any member of the audience's view, and just gently waft their veils to form a sort of background and ambience; no intricate veil movements, just gentle wafts. Afterwards I asked the audience whether the veils in the background had been irritating and distracting. They told me it had added colour and movement and had not been distracting. So I shall continue to use that 'prop'.

Zaïda's Jacarandas (all in their 60's) have danced many times since that first performance and even did a double show where we were asked to dance in two different lounges at the same Nursing Home, so that more of the residents could watch. By the end of the second show (each about 30 minutes), the Jacarandas were saying they could 'go' another round. This shows how fit and enthusiastic they are.

It is DANCE. It is FUN. Why take it so seriously?

Zaïda

Student Feedback:

"Taking into consideration our age group—I feel it is a most enjoyable way to exercise, which produces great 'side effects'—viz—tones up the body—reshapes the body—produces happiness and is good for the soul.

There is nothing more boring than to attend a gym regularly—with all those passive exercise machines.

Although some moves seem complicated, I find it does 'all come together' eventually with dedication and practice—and taking things at one's own pace,. The music and dancing are great for 'losing oneself' and shaking off any inhibitions which can hinder one from enjoyment.

I enjoy the warm up exercises better now, since more have been added. Also, I feel good being able to 'isolate' different parts of the body. (I seldom need pain killers these days and am positive Mondays *(class day)* have helped tremendously).

Veil work is most enjoyable and I tend to get lost in it. I feel I would like a longer class time and to spend more time on movements to increase my repertoire.

I do not like the connotation many people put on belly dancing and am forever explaining that we are 'classy' not 'sleazy'. You cannot compare an apple and an orange and the way one dances is personal. We all interpret things differently and are affected differently by the music. For me, it is a great way to lift the spirit and to relax and I certainly have never felt so well.

They say 'Life Begins At Forty'.... well, I reckon it begins at **SIXTY**!"

"I was looking for exercise, or simply folk dance classes (Greek or Israeli); and I found Belly Dance!

As long as classes remain fun with gentle pressure to achieve an expected level of expertise, they will be attractive to our age group....

which RULES out competition, but doesn't mean we won't try to improve.

Personally, I also find the history and background interesting."

CHAPTER 4

DANCING

'Achievement is largely the product of steadily raising one's level of aspiration and expectation'.

You will become so enthusiastic over your newfound passion that you will be unable to stop yourself telling anyone who'll listen, all about belly dancing.

This will lead to invitations to dance at parties and gatherings of your peers—especially women's groups and fundraising efforts or Homes for the Aged.

These groups are very appreciative of any entertainment and will support you wholeheartedly when they see how much you are enjoying yourself. At each party or gathering you will receive a number of enquiries about how to learn. You will have a 'party piece', which really makes them sit up and take notice.

I have been told again and again, that I look like a sixteen year old when I dance. For a 65 year old woman, this is unbelievable......but I BELIEVE, because that is how I FEEL!

Remember, if nobody was prepared to entertain his or her peers, life would be very dull.

Choose the places where you will perform, very carefully, and you will never receive any unpleasant responses from your audiences.

Aged person's homes and hostels, respite care facilities, club functions for older people, charity fund-raisers, private family celebrations—all these are fun places to dance.

I danced at a '***Virtual Flight***', which was a fundraiser, variety concert. The audience were 'travelling by aeroplane' and each time they 'landed' some form of entertainment, pertinent to that country, was provided.

For example, in Scotland there was a piper, in Ireland there were Irish Dancers, in the Philippines there were Filipina dancers, in Hawaii there was a Hula Dancer, in France a Can Can Dancer, a Didgeridoo player in Australia, a male opera singer in Italy, at the North Pole we met Santa Claus, and so on. I represented Egypt, and as I glided off stage, past the pilots, one pilot said to me, "You can do that AGAIN', so I guess he enjoyed my dance.

The two 'pilots' were the emcees and they were absolutely hilarious as they were discussing a lady passenger and the 'hostess' rushed into their mock-up flight deck and told them their P.A. microphone was switched on.

Then one of the pilots climbed out of the aircraft, in mid-flight, to clean the windscreen.

The hostesses gave an excruciatingly funny demonstration of the safety procedures in the event of a crash. During the 'flight' they served little nibblies/finger food pertinent to each of the countries they were about to visit.

This was a night to remember and the audience immersed themselves in the atmosphere, pretending they were on an actual flight.

When you feel confident about dancing before an audience, you may like to select an exotic name, as your dancing persona. It certainly adds to your performance to be introduced as Sheherezade rather than Jane. If you are looking for an Arabic name, your Library may be able to help with your search, or if you do not 'surf' cyber space, you can ask a friend who is active on the Internet, to type into the Search box, 'Arabic Names' and you will be swamped with sites containing names—and sometimes, their meanings.

Enjoy your dancing and your audience will enjoy watching.

If you are in a studio situation, you may find you have to dance in a sort of 'chorus line'. This is, unfortunately, necessary due to time constraints. It is just not possible to give each dancer a solo spot; if there are a number of dancers.

Belly dancing is not a chorus-line dance such as Riverdance. Its charm lies in the self-expression of each dancer. Each dancer moves differently and there is none of the rigidity found in classical dance such as ballet, where a certain move HAS to be done in a certain way. Ballet dancers even have to conform to a certain body type, but this does not apply to Belly Dancers. Each dancer interprets the music and the various moves in her own way, and body shape is of no consequence whatsoever.

A classic example of this, is the interpretation of 'THE CAMEL'.

This is a very simple, basic move, where you imagine you have a hinge just below your ribs. You do a figure eight on this hinge. Imagine someone has given you a sharp poke in the small of your back causing you to move your spine forward, and then a sharp poke in your belly button causing you to shrink your belly upwards and backwards. With practice you will develop an undulation.

If you do an opposite figure eight, this is 'The Fish' or reverse Camel.

You can layer this basic move in any way you wish, with arms, legs, head, feet, shimmies, walking, travelling, anything at all, but the basic Camel remains the same.

Because there has been so much discussion over this particular movement, I have done a great deal of research and asked several teachers for their input and I have gleaned that they all do the basic Camel, but add their own embellishments.

THE SHIMMY

This is the most complex movement to LEARN, but the easiest to do, once it is mastered. You will find yourself shimmying at the most unexpected moments.... to warm yourself if you are feeling cold...as a displacement activity when you are irritated waiting in a queue or for service…or just for the sheer joy of it.

To learn the shimmy, stand with feet slightly apart and drum your heels on the floor. Feel the movement in your hips and thighs, and register that feeling. This is not the correct way to shimmy, it is merely a means of learning how it should feel.

Once you become more flexible, you will shimmy merely by pushing your thigh muscles forward and back, very rapidly.

Later you may add other movements to your shimmy; like figure eights, circles, hip flicks, etc.

Zaïda's SHIMMY

Start your shimmy at the hips, let it imperceptibly move up to the chest, then as imperceptibly to the head, then back down again. As the shimmy leaves the hips, the hips become stationary and the movement is all in the chest, then the chest becomes stationary and only the head moves. This will take a bit of practice to get the isolations and to get the flow of the movement so that is becomes almost an undulation. Very effective and always produces a gasp from the audience.

YOUR SOLO

The chorus-line is not a part of belly dancing. You may be dancing with a group of women, but this is not the same as the 'chorus-line' of Western style dancing. Each woman would be interpreting the music to suit her own personality and physique.

So try to dance as a solo artist, perhaps with a friend, then you can work up a program of alternating solos with, possibly a duet at the end, but with each dancer interpreting the music in her own style. This looks truly beautiful and is a very effective closure to a performance.

To work up your own solo, you first need to select a tune, preferably one which has a number of changes of tempo, pace, colour, feel to the music. Become totally familiar with your selected tune by playing it every time you are doing a moronic chore, like ironing. Slowly the tune will sink into your subconscious and you will anticipate the changes.

Next, you start to put moves to the different moods of the music. Highlight special phrases of the music. For instance, in my newest solo, there is one point where a pipe plays alone, no other instrument, for several bars; I dance, pretending I am holding, and playing, a long, thin pipe pointing up to the skies. The audience can imagine whatever instrument they like.

Also, in a couple of places the music is bouncy, and sharp drum cracks sound a bit like clapping, so I dance pretending to clap my hands together. This may or may not get the audience clapping. Depends on their mood.

At another point in the tune, the music goes completely silent for two beats. I frame my eyes with my hands, for a heartbeat.

Your solo will slowly take shape as you decide which moves fit the music. The best part about doing a solo, is that you can change it in the blink of an eye and nobody will know you have forgotten what you originally planned to do. You will find that you change your dance to suit the different energy levels of the different audiences. Sometimes you are fluid and graceful. Sometimes you are bouncy and cheeky. Yet it is basically the same dance. It is YOUR solo, so you can do what you like with it.

I once got a standing ovation. ::Hah Hah:: Everybody was already standing up to go home and the emcee asked them all to thank me, once more, for my dance. So they did, enthusiastically, so I can honestly say I got a standing ovation.

VEILS

Veils are part of the mystique of Middle Eastern Dance and are as diverse as the costuming.

Beginners usually opt for chiffon veils, as they are cheap to buy, but these are very limp and they soon become dissatisfied with the 'flow' of the veil.

My personal preference is for a veil twice my height, measuring from shoulder height to the ground. I like a 'crisp' veil so that it has a lot of 'snap' for fast movements, so I use Pearl Organza. For a while I used veils made from Crystal Organza, but my newest veil is Pearl Organza and I am much happier with this veil as it is softer than the Crystal and thus easier to drape, but is still lovely and crisp.

Many dancers like Silk. I have never danced with a silk veil and so cannot comment, but I feel they would lend themselves more to the slow, sultry movements or draping of the body.

You need to consider your style of dancing when choosing your veil.

It is best not to have any attachments to the veil as they just may catch your eye as you dance and I mean, literally.

Most veils are almost transparent to allow body movements to be seen through the veil, but you can use an opaque veil, if that is your preference.

There are no hard and fast rules, so make your own decisions.

Some veil movements are described in Chapter 9—Interesting Moves.

SWORDS—some dancers enjoy dancing with a sword. This can look very spectacular, but is not for every dancer…it is a personality thing.

If you like the sword, you can obtain finely crafted, perfectly balanced, lightweight, blunt swords, designed purely for dancing and made from stainless steel or bronze. These may be obtained from a true swordsmith, who has studied the history and the art of manufacture, then had his swords 'road tested' by a professional dancer who loves to dance with swords.

ZENOBIA PTAH AUSTRALIA
P.O. Box 1181 CALOUNDRA QLD 4551 AUSTRALIA
Phone in Australia 07 5494 6702F—Phone International +61 7 5494
6702

CUSTOM MADE SWORDS by Al Massey
email: armjan@attcanada.ca
Site 16 Box 14 RR#2, Mount Uniacke, Nova Scotia, BON IZO,
CANADA
Balanced dance swords.
Replicas—Medieval, Celtic, Roman, Scottish—Sgian Dubh, Dirks,
Claymore (a la Braveheart).
Hand forged Damascus steel.
Ideal for historic re-enactments or historical sites.

REMINDER: ALWAYS spend at least 10 minutes warming-up before
you start your dance. This not only protects your muscles but will ensure
that your body is fluid and graceful when you START to dance and not
just when you have been dancing for a while.

Warming-up may seem unnecessary when you are all hyped-up and
'hot-to-trot'. In fact it can even seem a tiresome waste of time, but it is
VERY important—if you want to dance to the best of your ability.

Warming up is telling your body that it is about to dance and stretching your muscles and ligaments so they are flexible. It also gets your mind
focused.

CHAPTER 5

MUSIC

'Work like you don't need the money;
Love like you've never been hurt;
Dance like nobody's watching'

Westerners, with their passion for order have devolved a musical scale, which has equal intervals between notes. This is the sound to which our ears have become attuned since birth.

Middle Eastern music uses a microtonic scale which incorporates intervals smaller than a semitone. This can sound quite discordant to the Western ear, until that ear is trained to accept the new tonic scale.

The musical scale, the 7 major notes, corresponds to the 7 main colours, red through purple, and these correspond to the 7 chakra or energy centres in the body, from the sacrum (sacred bone = pelvic vertebrae) to the top of the head.

This is why music is the last 'sense' to be lost in cases of dementia. Many people can still SING even after losing their ability to speak. It has been observed that people in Nursing Homes, who appear to be completely unaware, will respond to music. Music has proven to be beneficial to animals as well, and many dairy farmers have pleasant music (at bovine heartbeat tempo) playing during milking.

Music is used as a calming device in places like lifts, where people may become tense; or as an atmosphere generator in street marches and pageants.

Music is such an integral part of our BEING, that we respond to music without even realising it. Hear a guitar being strummed on a street corner

41

and your antennae immediately seek out the source of the sound. Music is used in all aspects of human life and reaches our very core. Even people who claim to have a 'tin' ear will respond to marching bands; and the most pleasing music is that which is played at a beat which is the same tempo as our heart-beat. This is why 'background' music is used to set the mood in films and will slow down or speed up according to the mood the film maker wishes to instil.

Many dancers prefer Westernised music. Some even dance to modern pop music. This is within the nature of the dance. After all, the dance was originally the dance of the ordinary people and they danced to their ordinary music—'pop music'—before the term was invented. You dance to whatever music works for you. My personal preference is for the Arabic sound which has been Westernised, enough not to be discordant to my ear but has not lost the Arabic 'feel'—the complicated rhythms without the high-pitched wailing sounds. I also tend to avoid vocals, because I have no idea what is being expressed..... and could easily misinterpret a song, thus truly annoying anyone who can understand the words. Worse, I could be really offensive without realising it.

Also, it is necessary to consider the tastes of your audience. If you are dancing for a Western audience, they will not appreciate pure Middle Eastern/Arabic music. If you are dancing for an Arabic audience, then they would prefer their traditional sound.

Middle Eastern music is based on extremely complex rhythms and this is what gives it the rich texture, which makes your feet want to dance. You cannot listen to belly dance music and not want to dance. Even audiences who are experiencing this dance for the first time are carried away by the intricate and compelling rhythms. You will see feet tapping and swinging and fingers rapping, but most importantly, you will see smiles.... lots of smiles. Middle Eastern music is HAPPY music.

In the ninth century a musician named Ziryab, migrated from Baghdad to Cordoba in Spain; he felt too stifled by the traditionalists in his country who insisted the music must be played 'correctly'.

Ziryab exerted enormous influence on Moorish Spain and the music and instruments of the East were quickly absorbed into European culture. Spanish Flamenco dancing and guitar style is a well-known and popular, outcome of this exchange of ideas.

For new dancers still searching for their particular style, I recommend Emad Sayyah's collection of CD's titled 'Modern Belly Dance From Lebanon'. My favourite is the double CD set called '*The Night is Beautiful*'. I must admit I have not heard **all** his CD's, but this is the pick of the ones I have heard. My main criticism is that he has about 50% vocals, and many Western dancers avoid vocals due to the fact that they have no idea what the singer is singing about and don't want to take the risk of fitting the wrong dance to the sense of the song. Also, Western audiences seem to prefer the music only selections.

Your choice of music is as individual as your choice of costume and dance style. You must feel the music 'move' you. Some dancers like bright and energetic, others prefer mysterious sounds. You will know your tune when you hear it, and the only way to find it is to listen and listen and listen, because it takes a while for the music to 'speak' to you. Your ear has to first become accustomed to this style of music.

I am teaching a small group of older women the sheer JOY of belly dance. At first, they all said the music sounded the same and I had to signal to them when to change from one movement to another. For me, this spoilt the flow of the dance.

Suddenly, one day they all changed direction at exactly the right moment and I felt such a thrill. They were finally HEARING the music.

I dislike having the dancers count their steps, as that way they do not respond to the nuances of the music. Once they can HEAR the music, they will interpret it according to their own feelings. Thus, there may be several dancers all dancing to the same tune, but they will be dancing their own, individual dances. I just get them to join together for short chorus segments, where they are all doing the same thing, but not in strict, regimented unison. The colour, the movement, the sheer exuberance of the dancers create JOY.

Several get so lost in the dance, that they forget all about the 'chorus' sections, and that is lovely, as it proves they are totally immersed in the dance and the music. They forget to be self-conscious and have complained at the end of the tune, that 'it was not long enough'.

As you progress with your dancing, you will find tunes, which you previously by-passed are now attracting your attention; so initially, wait until you enjoy listening to a particular tune. As you become more proficient, you will think of moves which will fit previously complicated sounding tunes. You might have thought a tune much too fast, but as you become accustomed to the rhythms, you will realise you do not have to dance at the speed of the melody...you can dance to the bass percussion, interspersed with dancing to the melody. You can also use quieter spells to 'have a rest' by using only arm movements for a few bars.

My personal preference is for tunes which have frequent changes of tempo, style, shading and emotion. This keeps you interested, but more importantly, keeps your audience interested.

Dance without music would be a non-event and would be totally boring for the dancer and for the audience.

Music is the core of our existence.

CHAPTER 6

SALUBRITY

'Conducive or favourable to health or well-being'

You will find yourself moving with more fluidity when you walk and the stiffness which was hampering your life, will be gone. You will walk with a 'spring' in your step and will be able to squat down to talk with someone sitting in a wheelchair, and then stand up again without effort. You will lose your fear of stairs or rough surfaces. Perhaps, you will even be able to jump once more. Little jumps, like over a puddle.

All the movements used in Belly Dancing are designed to strengthen the muscles and improve flexibility. In doing these movements, the muscles work on the internal organs of the body and improve their performance.

The spine is given greater flexibility, as strengthening the abdominal and side muscles protects the back, where the muscles in the small of the back are particularly thin and weak.

Sessions start with deep breathing and stretching the body upwards to give the lungs greater capacity. Breathing into the abdomen gives the lungs more space to work and allows all that stale air accumulated at the bottom of the lungs, to be expelled. When you breathe out deeply, you automatically breathe in, just as deeply.

Arm and leg muscles are stretched and relaxed to improve flexibility and the neck is flexed in every direction except backwards; **never** backwards, this can be extremely dangerous. The muscles which hold the shoulders and hips in their correct positions, are strengthened, thus reducing risk of injury to the sockets.

Over a period of time, the weight of the head tends to drag the neck muscles forward and without constant flexing these muscles weaken—thus the 'dowager's hump' makes an appearance. Also, the modern addiction to computers tends to bring the head forward on the neck and this posture is sure to trigger health problems.

Balance is improved as the leg muscles strengthen and knee, ankle and hip flexibility improves. You will find you no longer need to grasp handrails when descending stairs. You will be far less liable to slip and fall on uneven surfaces. You will feel much safer in the bath or shower.

Shoulders are stretched and flexed until the shoulders are completely free and can move independently through a wide arc of movement; (Westerners tend not to move their shoulders very much, thus they seize up and this can be the cause of headaches).

The rib cage is moved sideways, forwards, backwards and in diamond and circle configurations whilst keeping the remainder of the body completely stationary. Loosening up the rib cage allows for much deeper breathing capacity.

Then the hips are moved through the same movements whilst keeping the rib cage stationary. Hip movements cover an extremely wide range and incorporate flicks and drops and sits and figure eights (which can be horizontal, forward and back, or vertical).

Circles are drawn with the hips without moving the rest of the torso—little circles and big circles. Circles can also involve moving the rib cage in a counter-balancing circle to the hips.

A stress reducing hip circle involves making very small hip circles whilst holding the hands above the head with the hands facing forward, one hand in the palm of the other. Make tiny hip circles and breathe deeply. This is an excellent movement to make just prior to going to bed to sleep.

Abdominal muscles are flexed in circular movements upwards, sideways and obliquely, creating abdominal rolls, flutters and waves.

Abdominal muscle movements allow all the internal abdominal organs to receive a beneficial massage, particularly the intestines. A gentle warning—if you do belly rolls for more than a couple of minutes, you may end up with a case of diarrhoea.

All these movements are performed whilst moving the arms, feet, neck, shoulders, even eyes and eyelids. This is called 'layering'.

LYMPH

When muscles stretch and contract they stimulate the many vital organs within the torso as well as the lymph system. Elimination of toxic substances within the body will be markedly enhanced by the stimulation of the lymph system. The manipulation of the abdominal muscles creates a massage effect on the major lymph tract, which runs up the centre of the torso to the top of the rib cage, where toxic lymph is discharged into the venous system and thus eliminated from the body.

Exercise decreases blood volumes in venous reservoirs such as the spleen. The shifts in reservoirs makes more blood available to the heart, arteries and exercising muscle, and respiration becomes more efficient. The body learns to mobilise sources of nutrients rapidly for energy production.

GRAVITY

21st Century scientific observations of Astronauts who have spent extended periods of time in Space, have shown that in a gravity-free environment there is considerable loss of calcium, bone density and muscle mass.

Astronauts may take several years to recover their pre-flight health status.

The conclusion is that it is vital to constantly 'resist' gravity in order to remain healthy. Therefore, it is better for you to climb those stairs, resisting gravity all the way, than to take the lift. It is better for you to get up out of that chair instead of asking the children 'or hubby', to bring you cups of tea.

Resisting gravity is the best way to keep your body healthy and negate the expected effects of ageing.

MUSCLES

There are two general types of muscle in the body—cardiac and skeletal.

Skeletal muscles fall into two general types, commonly known as 'fast twitch' or white muscle and 'slow twitch' or red muscle. 'Fast twitch' are responsible for rapid, sudden movements, whilst 'slow twitch' maintain slower, sustained movements. Individuals are born with a set ratio of 'fast twitch' muscles to 'slow twitch' muscles and this ratio is unchangeable. However, the ratio of these muscles in **individual** body parts does vary from person to person.

Thus athletes with a higher ratio of 'fast twitch' muscles in their legs will make good sprinters, whereas those athletes with a higher ratio of 'slow twitch' muscles in their legs will make good marathon runners.

For this reason dancers will perform movements totally differently each from the other. This makes the individualistic style of belly dancing most appealing; there is no demand to conform to a rigid structure.

To become a classical ballet dancer, you need to have a specific build; you need to have a specific number of 'fast twitch' and 'slow twitch' muscles in a specific proportion in a specific area of the body.

To become a belly dancer, there is no restriction on weight, height, age or eye colour.

Dancers progress at their own speed and ability and are not pressured into performing at a level of activity beyond their comfort zone. A move, which is impossible one week, will suddenly 'happen' the next week. Your muscles have to be taught to move in unfamiliar ways and it often takes a sleep period for the brain to register and 'save' a new movement.

SPECIFIC HEALTH BENEFITS

Doctors are now recommending belly dancing as a pain management system for women suffering from Endometriosis. Blood pressure is stabilised, the heart muscle is strengthened, lung capacity increased and the whole body is left with a feeling of well-being.

Fertility is enhanced and a dancer can expect a trouble free pregnancy and birthing. It was customary for dancers to dance around a woman in labour. This took her mind off her discomfort and set the mood for a joyous occasion. As the labour progressed the music became more driving and the dancing increased in tempo. Often the woman in labour would rise and dance for a short while. This kept her body flexible and her muscles strong.

Symptoms of post-natal depression do not get a chance to establish themselves when dancers resume their dancing as soon as they hear the music. Childbirth is not an illness, but a natural process and dancing complements that natural process.

One lady, a midwife, suffering from agoraphobia after the birth of her son, found that bellydancing helped her to regain her self-confidence; as her agility improved she was able to leave her 'comfort zone' and resume her life.

A dancer, born with hip dysplasia, found that as her muscles strengthened, her hip would stay in place for longer and longer periods, the last episode occurring more than a year after the previous episode.

SENSUALITY > 'affecting any of the senses'

It is important not to confuse 'sensuality' with 'sexuality'.

Dancers find that they feel more confident and worthwhile. They also become much more sensual women. They are more comfortable with their own bodies and their emotions. They can express previously suppressed emotions, thus allowing themselves to 'feel'.

Dancers' spouses are the most enthusiastic supporters of this form of dance. After a Belly Dance session, dancers are on a 'high' and ready to 'party'. Many dancers report that after their early dance lessons, they were unable to sleep; their minds and bodies were totally hyped-up. Later, as their fitness improved they found that they dropped into a deep slumber when they retired after a dance session.

Dancers walk with a grace and balance they never knew could be theirs. They tread lightly along their pathway of life. Dancing becomes more important than many pointless concerns. Dancing is a special, health-giving philosophy of life.

A dancer will probably take about 6 months to reach a good standard of flexibility, muscle power and balance; but even the first lesson will be fun, with much laughter and happy feelings.

BRAIN-WASHING

Western dancers have to overcome their rigid upbringing, to forget the doctrines drummed into them as children, 'Don't show off your bust. Don't wiggle your bottom. Don't draw attention to yourself. Don't!'

Often this is a long, hard grind. Brain-washing in the first 7 years of life is likely to be set in concrete and it takes a jack-hammer to break that concrete setting. Belly dancing is a very efficient jack-hammer in this situation. The dance becomes more important than your parents' hang-ups, which were probably merely a mindless continuation of **their** parents' hang-ups.

Dancers are encouraged to learn hip circles and rib circles. This breaks the mind-set that 'you don't move that part of your body'. Indeed, many Western women are totally immobile through the entire torso.

Flexibility is as much mental as physical. Tiny movements will grow into big movements as the brain allows the body to move; but once you learn that there is no embarrassment in moving the body and come to love the driving music, you will become an enthusiast.

YOU WILL DANCE!

CHAPTER 7

$\mathcal{STAMINA}\ \&$
$\mathcal{FLEXIBILITY}$

"Wine, Women and Cheese all improve with age"

Check with your doctor
before starting any exercise program
Warning! If you experience pain—STOP!
Do not eat a meal within two hours prior to dancing

BREATHING is the most important aspect of dancing. Correct breathing improves stamina, health, vitality and the sheer joy of being alive.

Breathe from the abdomen. Your ribs are fairly rigid, so you need to allow your lungs to SPREAD downwards, thus emptying and replenishing the lower part of the lungs with fresh oxygen. Inhale long, slow, deep breaths, but not so deep as to hyperventilate and become giddy. Practice breathing from the abdomen until it becomes automatic. A few seconds at a time, whenever you think about it; the seconds will mount to minutes, then hours. As your breathing improves so will your sense of well-being. Oxygenating your blood encourages self-healing in all areas and organs of the body. Correct breathing will prevent many minor illnesses from becoming major calamities, by assisting the body to rout out the intruders and repair the damage. Correct breathing creates a flow of *'life-force'* throughout the body and is a major component in ancient traditions like Yoga and Tai Chi.

Expand your ribs. Expand your abdomen. Expand your life.

WARM UP

(Here in the tropics, beginners often say "I am already warm", so perhaps a better phrase would be LOOSEN UP).

An excellent warm-up exercise, before dancing, incorporates correct breathing. I stand with my feet the same distance apart as my hip bones, knees slightly flexed and relaxed. Pelvis is tilted backward (bum tucked under) to straighten the small of the back and tone the abdominal muscles. This is called the Pelvic Tilt and is the absolute basis of belly dancing. You cannot dance with a slouch. You cannot dance with a hollow back.

PELVIC TILT

Pelvic tilt improves posture and reduces lower-back stress. Learn this position lying down. Concentrate on how your spine feels, the position of your hips and the tension in your muscles, then maintain this position when upright. Practice will make it automatic—you will be unable to stand any other way.

Lie on your back with knees bent. Press the hollow in the small of your back onto the floor. Tighten abdominal and buttock muscles, then raise buttocks slightly off the floor, maintaining the pressure of the lower back against the floor. Hold for 14 seconds. Repeat three times. Take note of how your body feels when in this position and try to recapture that feeling once you are standing upright. Reminding yourself to tilt your pelvis, whenever you think of it, will make the stance second nature and you will find yourself uncomfortable in your old slouch. The pelvic tilt will reduce or even eliminate backache, especially when you find you have to stand for some considerable period of time. Pelvic Tilt is not a matter of 'sucking-in' your abdominal muscles—it is a definite straightening of the spine at the pelvis.

BACK TO THE WARM UP......

Start with the hands held out to the sides, palms down. On a slow in-breath through the nostrils, bring the hands downwards to the hips, inwards to the front of the pelvis where one hand is in front of the other, both facing towards the body. Bring the hands up the centre of the body. Turn the hands outwards at the chakra (about heart level) pushing up above the head with palms facing upwards but one hand still cupped in the other.

On the out-breath through the mouth open the arms out sideways and lowering in a downward arc with the fingers pointing upwards, palms facing outwards, allowing the base of the palm (the heel of the hand) to lead the hand (another chakra).

The exercise is reversed after four breaths. With palms facing down, on an in-breath slowly raise the hands sideways away from the body in an upward arc, until they are above the head. Fingers remain gently relaxed pointing to the ground, until hands reach the apex. This bent, relaxed position activates the energy point at the back of the wrist (chakra). At the apex fingers point directly upward with the thumbs horizontal. Both hands face forward, the back of one hand in the palm of the other (hands of Fatima).

On a slow out-breath through the mouth bring hands down the centre of the body, turning on the chakra (energy point in the heart region) so that palms face up, and back to the start position.

This exercise will improve your breathing, your health and help to stretch the torso to increase flexibility.

Join the fingers of both hands together in front of your body. Breathe in and bring both hands together up the centre of the body, turning on the chakra, then right up above your head, keeping fingers joined (palms are now facing upwards). Raise up on tiptoe. Breathe out as backs of joined hands lower to touch the top of your head, lowering your weight onto your heels. Then stretch up again onto your toes on an in-breath, the hands remain joined and this will flex the wrists backwards; breathe out as hands lower to top of head, and your weight lowers onto your heels. Do the stretch up, and head touching bit 4 times.

FLEXIBLE SPINE—Stand with feet slightly apart, facing forward. Let the upper body twist to the right with the arms flopping loosely. Twist as far round as you can without discomfort. Return to the front and twist to the left. Repeat several times, keeping your arms as floppy as possible. Let your eyes move as far around the arc as possible; very good eye exercise. Remember to **keep the hips still** or the twist will not be in your waist, but in your knees, and you will find you have sore knees.

Remember the Pelvic Tilt.

Stand facing forward and hold both hands in front at shoulder level, with fists **lightly** closed. Twist to the right keeping the fists in front of the shoulders. Twist as far as possible without discomfort. Twist back to the front then twist to the left. Repeat several times. Gently. Keep your hips still to safeguard your knees.

Remember the Pelvic Tilt.

Both hands by your sides, stretch one hand straight up, arm straight, as high above your head as you can reach. Allow the other hand to do what it will. Change hands and stretch the other side. FEEL that pull all down your side; your aim is to stretch those side, waist muscles. 4 repeats each side.

A good spine flexing movement is to stand in your start position, arms straight up above your head. Grasp your right wrist with your left hand and bend sideways to the left, making sure you do not bend forwards or backwards. The aim is to stretch the spine **sideways**. Pull your right arm as far over to the left as you can, without pain. You will feel a stretch all the way down your right hand side. It may help to stand with your feet slightly further apart. Repeat on the other side by holding the left wrist with the right hand and bending to the right, pulling the left wrist and stretching the left side. GENTLY.

Spread your feet further apart, bend the left knee and lean to the left with your left elbow resting on your left knee and your right arm reaching over your head to form a curve to the left. Stretch your right leg out sideways as far as is comfortable. You will feel a stretch right up your right-hand side. Slowly change to a squat and swing both arms to the front with the knees still in the squat position, work on achieving a DEEP squat (Western women suffer a number of health problems simply because they never SQUAT), then rest your right elbow on your right knee, straighten your left knee sideways and your left arm makes a curve over your head to the right. You will feel a stretch right up your left-hand side. 4 repeats on both sides.

Squat and stretch both hands straight out in front of the body, with your body bent forwards so that your head is between your elbows. Straighten up and grasp your hands behind your back whilst pushing your hips forward. This will help to free up your hips. 4 repeats.

STIFFNESS—take a lesson from your cat. Position yourself on your hands and knees with hands at shoulder width and knees about 20cm apart. Slowly raise your head to look up at the sky, push your bottom up and outward, curving your back as if you were to push your stomach towards the floor. Very gently. Hold for 7 seconds.

Return to start position; slowly drop your head between your upper arms, arching your back upwards into a curve. Hold for 7 seconds. Repeat exercise twice. GENTLY.

NECKS—NEVER tilt your neck BACKWARDS. Very dangerous!

Lower your left ear to your left shoulder and gently roll your chin down to your chest then your right ear to your right shoulder. Reverse. DO NOT tilt the head backwards—very risky. Ensure that your shoulders remain relaxed.

Slowly turn the head to look over the left shoulder, allow your eyes to follow through and look as far as possible to the left; then the right shoulder, then left, then right. A few of these turns will loosen the neck over a period of time; and strengthen the eye muscles. You may hear creaks and groans and clicks as your neck loosens up.

This is only NOISE.

Draw a circle with your chin. Imagine you have a pencil attached to your chin and are drawing circles on a piece of paper just under your chin.

4 circles one way, then 4 the other.

Head bobs forward and back.

The Crescent is done by moving the chin in a crescent shape across the front of the body. As the chin rises to the right, the eyes go to the left and upwards. The chin comes down and across in a crescent shape and the eyes go to the right and upwards.

SHOULDERS—Move your shoulders forward and back, independently.

Lift shoulders up to your ears and drop them to normal position. Roll shoulders in a circle with the arm hanging down the side of the body. The circle is forward, up to the roof, backward, down to the floor—a vertical circle. Do this forwards and backwards a few times with each shoulder.

Hold your arm out straight in front of your body and circle the shoulder. Concentrate on that ball rolling in the cup of your shoulder. The ARM does not move, or bend, or flap. Imagine that ball in your shoulder joint rolling around in the cup into which it fits. All the movement is in the shoulder. Reverse that roll. 4 times each way and repeat with the other arm. If you feel pain...**STOP!**

Arms straight down by your sides. Raise the right arm out sideways and continue until it is straight up above your head. Bring that arm down and raise the other. Flexing the wrists so that the heel of the hand is leading the hand downwards, (another energy chakra).

Remember your Pelvic Tilt.

Hold both arms straight out in front of you and give your hands a tiny circle to the left, then a larger circle, then the biggest circle you can manage, but only moving the wrists. Then repeat to the right…. this stimulates the Lymph system.

Fold your right arm over your left shoulder with the hand hanging down your back (slightly). Give that elbow a slight push with your left hand. Don't force it, just gentle pressure. Repeat other side. 2 repeats each side.

Reach your left arm up behind your back to between your shoulder blades. Reach your right arm over your shoulder down your back to join the fingers of the left hand. Repeat other side. Only do this once each side. May take a while before you can connect your fingers and don't force it or rush it. One day it will happen. If you feel PAIN…. STOP!

HIPS—Improving the flexibility of your hips, will improve your balance and your safety when walking, especially on uneven surfaces or when descending stairs. Your hips act like the shock absorbers and stabilisers in a motor car, levelling out the uneven surfaces and keeping your body on an even keel. The more flexibility in your hips, the better they stabilise your body.

Keeping the upper body still, but relaxed, move the hips to the right side as far as they will comfortably go. Return to mid-line and move hips to the left. Repeat cycle 4 times.

Make a figure eight with your hips by circling the right hip then the left hip. Imagine that figure eight. Start by taking the first hip backwards, then reverse this move, by taking the first hip forwards. 4 repeats in each direction.

Make a vertical figure eight by bringing the right hip upwards then down and then the left hip. Imagine that figure eight. Reverse this by taking the right hip downwards, then the left hip. 4 repeats in each direction.

You will find there is very little movement in your hips, at first, but keep picturing the move and suddenly, one day, you will find it HAPPENING.

After a childhood of being told to keep our hips still, it is not an easy matter to overcome those years of brainwashed, self-imposed rigidity.

CHESTS—Moving your chest is even more difficult than moving your hips, because of the same imposed rigidity. Make a circle with your rib cage, then reverse the circle. 4 times each way.

Chest drops, imagine someone is pulling your breast-bone upwards with a string and suddenly releasing it.

Chest lifts, imagine you are bouncing a 'ping-pong' ball upwards, with your chest.

Imagine you have two tassels attached to the front of your charms (if the image amuses you) and try to swing those tassels in a circle.

KINESIOLOGY—teaching the right brain (artistic) to talk to the left brain (logic). Always start these exercises to the **LEFT** as that means the right brain is leading.

Hold your arms out to the sides at shoulder level, so that your thumbs, held upright, are just within your peripheral vision on either side.

Starting to the LEFT—ALWAYS to the left, first, as this causes the right side of the brain to lead, make a figure eight with your eyes, connecting both thumbs. 4 repeats.

Touch your left shoulder with your right hand and your nose with your left hand. Touch your thighs with both hands.

Touch your right shoulder with your left hand and your nose with your right hand. Touch your thighs with both hands.

The hand touching your nose is always OUTSIDE the hand touching your shoulder. Do this as **FAST** as you possibly can. 4 repeats of cycle.

Remember the Pelvic Tilt.

Lunge forward with right foot, but keeping the left HEEL on the floor, behind you. Keep the rear foot facing forwards and do not allow it to turn outwards—this will put tension on the calf muscles in that leg. Hold this position for 8 heartbeats. This move will stretch the calf and thigh muscles. Repeat with the other leg. Once each side.

If you feel PAIN.... **STOP!**

Remember the Pelvic Tilt.

BALANCE—stand on tiptoes and stretch to the roof. You may need to start this exercise whilst standing under an archway so that you can stretch and still have something to hold onto. In time, you will not need support and will be able to stand on tiptoe for some minutes. BELIEVE ME.... it will happen.

Stand with feet at hip width, pelvis tilted, and raise the right knee across the front of the body. Sweeping both hands together in a huge figure eight, sweep hands downwards past the outside of the right knee. Drop right knee and raise left knee forwards across the front of the body whilst the hands are on the upward sweep of the figure eight, then sweep the hands down on the outside of the left knee. Several, slow repetitions of this exercise will enhance your kinetic responses in your brain and improve your balance. The slower you can make this movement, the more you will benefit.

Stand with feet at hip width and raise arms sideways until they are horizontal. Raise the right knee and move it outwards until it points directly to your right, in the bent position. Make a figure eight with your right knee by bringing it across in front of your body and back out to the right side. Repeat on the left side. Several slow repetitions. Excellent for balance and for hip mobility.

Hip mobility is essential for balance when walking or descending stairs.

'GENTLY, GENTLY CATCHEE MONKEE'

All exercise must be gentle and not stress the body. Pain or stiffness will only make you reluctant to exercise. Do not try to push your body beyond its capabilities and you will find your limits stretch further and further as you become fitter and fitter.

A LITTLE GOES A LONG WAY

A short session of ten minutes, every day, is more beneficial for an older person, than one long session of thirty minutes, or more, twice a week. Establish a pattern so that you do not even think about it, but just get out of bed, put on your music and do your warm-up routine. Tell yourself it is only a couple of minutes, then you will not waste that few minutes thinking up an excuse NOT to exercise.

Once the music takes hold of you then it is no longer a chore. Muscle strength will improve and this will reduce the risk of injury. Taking your exercise slowly and gently—only increasing the pace as you feel comfortable in doing so—will not lead to ripped ligaments, popped tendons or torn muscles, as many people fear. You can do a short exercise whilst waiting for some machine to complete its job; such as the washing machine— or when sitting in your car at traffic lights……this is quite startling, especially the shoulder shimmy, for occupants of other cars; but do you **CARE?**

Exercise…. **any** exercise…. burns fat.

BACK PROBLEMS may be eased through regular use of gentle exercises. This exercise also improves flexibility: kneel on the floor; kneel on your right knee, move your left foot forward so that your shin makes a 60° angle to the floor. Your weight comes forward onto your left foot, push your right foot backwards onto the toes and then lower your torso so that your hands rest on the floor on each side of your left foot. Your back and outstretched right leg must remain in a straight line. Hold for 7 seconds. Return to start position, then repeat with opposite foot positions. Do twice on each side; **SLOWLY AND GENTLY.**

YOGA & TAI CHI

Arabic dance is a VERY ancient form of dance, and you will see many Yoga and Tai Chi moves in the dance. All these disciplines have copied from each other over the centuries, as people move around the world.

FLEXIBILITY IS IN THE MIND

Flexibility is as much controlled by the mind as by the fitness of the body. If you are 'uptight' and feel uncomfortable moving your body, then you will be stiff and rigid. Work on relaxing your mind. Change your mental attitude about using your body as a musical instrument. Tell yourself, you are the music and let yourself 'shape' the notes.

CONTINENCE

You will experience improved continence. This is commonly a problem for women who have given birth; especially if the baby was very large.

STAMINA

New dancers find that an hour lesson is far too long. They usually run out of 'puff' by the last fifteen minutes. As week follows week and they keep practicing, the hour will get shorter and shorter, and they may even feel they have been cheated and not given the full hour. This is STA-MINA.

ENJOY!

Enjoyment is the keyword. As you get stronger and fitter, so your enjoyment will escalate. Your energy will increase and you will want to DANCE!.

Just as clouds let you SEE air—so dance lets you SEE music.

Warning! If you experience pain—STOP!

Tension is not pain.
Creaking noise is not pain.
Stretching muscle is not pain.

CHAPTER 8

FOR MEN

by ANKH

It is rather difficult to define how Male belly dance differs from Female. There is no simple answer.

It is mostly a matter of body language, much as a Hula dancer tells a story, a Mid-Eastern dancer paints an image. Mid-Eastern dance in abstract is neither Feminine nor Masculine, but the body language we are used to seeing in the dance, is predominantly Feminine. The trick is to change the body language to Masculine.

In Egypt, not long ago, it was (and may still be) common for males and females to 'belly dance' as couples in Discos.

So how do I do that? This is where it becomes difficult to draw lines or make rules.

Take HAND MOTIONS—I suggest that a Male dancer avoid the 'limp wrist' look. This does not mean that a male should not do 'snake arms' or other similar moves that involve a supple wrist, but perhaps that a supple wrist should not be the focus except for a passing moment. It might be good for a Male dancer to stay off the toes a bit more than the ladies. A good trick is to choreograph dances with sections that have male and female parts, the female parts should lean toward smooth delicate motions of beauty (the Beauty—like a gazelle), the male parts should lean toward motions of power and grace (the Beast—think

69

LION). The contrast of these sections shows audiences that the dancers KNOW they are Male and Female.

Attitude has a lot to do with the perceived Masculinity of the dance. A shy, demure look is better suited for the Female dancers; a Male should lean more toward the suave and diviner look. Just as the Female dancer flirts with the male audience, veil over the head, etc. the Male dancer should flirt with the female audience. Just use good judgement, or some hubby/boyfriend could cause a nasty scene—nothing new there, except it is the wife or girlfriend who may blow up with the female dancer.

(comment by Zaïda.… 'I have seen a young woman, sitting with her arm draped softly across her man's shoulders, suddenly tighten her hold into a stranglehold around his neck, when I did a shoulder shimmy in front of them'.)

The dance costume should have a Manly look about it, bold colours, no pastels or washed out colours. Jewellery should be less dainty, perhaps of heavier construction.

Music is a major part of a dance performance, and for a solo Male dancer, should also reinforce in some way the Manliness of the performance. A stronger Beastlier beat is a good start. I would suggest staying away from delicate music, and go straight for the Industrial Strength Raqs Sharqi, or the like.

While putting it all together pay attention to the overall effect. If you could not tell the sex of the male dancer, could your audience mistake him for a female dancer? If so, what change would prevent that mistake? When layering motions, consider how they fit together, and whether that combination 'speaks' mostly in female body language.

Most important of all—GIVE IT A GO—and ENJOY the dance. You will never be able to please everyone, so don't sweat it. Be your own judge of what looks good on you and work at making it look all the better.

I suggest not avoiding learning any move that you think may not be Male enough, but rather learn the move, and if it doesn't feel right, don't use it. Instead, teach it to the ladies who are interested in learning the move. You may be surprised at what that move may change into later on.

My BEST WISHES to all the Dancers.

ENJOY.......**ANKH**

Ankh's Website....
http://hometown.aol.com/ANKHoISIS/index.html

Some more comments from **ANKH**
"Hey look at this, there is a GUY in this belly dance book!!".
"Yea what's he doing in there?"
Now that I have your attention, let me introduce myself. My dance name is Ankh, from the ancient Egyptian symbol of life. Yes I am a male Mid-Eastern dancer.

For several years now, I have been training, rehearsing and dancing as a member of a very large (around 300 dancers) and stable troupe (over 20 years) "Isis and the Star Dancers" based in Dallas / Fort Worth (Texas USA). I am in the studio 12 or more hours a week on the average and perform as the opportunity arises. I also participate in workshops and seminars as often as I am able.

The largest of these that I have had the pleasure to enjoy was Rakkasah West, a solid week of workshops and a weekend of endless performances. Rakkasah is quite amazing, I highly recommend it.

My primary dance form is "Mid-Eastern Dance" also known as "Belly Dance", with "Raks Sharki" or "Free Dancing" being one of my favourite flavours. As a troupe we also have group choreography including another of my favourite flavours "Mixed Couples" involving choreography distinctly for males and females.

I am also involved with "American Tribal", an interesting challenge as masculine males or costumes in this particular dance style seem to be non-existent.

What is masculine about "Belly Dance"? Hopefully not a thing—when a lady is dancing. However, when I dance, my primary focus is the females in the audience and my goal is to have the impact on them that a good female dancer has on the male audience.

Male and female dancers have a lot of common ground. A good dancer will dance the music, be confident, entertaining, and demonstrate a level of skill to be admired. All the basics of the dance form hold true for both male and female, the dance and the dance moves are a human thing not a gender thing. The difference is in the presentation. The female dancer is a projection of beauty; soft, bold, coy, seductive or dazzling as the mood of the music strikes her. The male dancer is a projection of strength, power, control, romance; he is the warrior; he is the MAN.

It is a matter of costuming, body language and most importantly attitude. The beautiful girl is a "babe" the handsome boy a "hunk".

Well it sounds good in theory at least, but how do you change effeminate dance into masculine dance? Lets take a simple example that has nothing to do with dance.

A gracious lady and a dashing man are introduced and are expected to shake hands. The lady offers her hand palm down with the wrist bent displaying the beauty of her hand, wrist and forearm. The man meets her hand palm to palm, softly but with implied strength, softly speaks a pleasantry and gracefully bows to kiss the back of her hand. The lady blushes, with a tittering giggle and hides her lower face with her fan.

In this example we have the contrast of the male and female intensified by the interaction of the two. How would it be if the male behaved just as the female in this encounter? Such is the way with the dance. It requires a bit of contrast in the male and female dance styles to remove the effeminate body language and attitude and replace it with the masculine.

Body language can be a very subtle thing, or can be quite obvious. Either way everyone reads it without even realizing it most of the time. This is especially true for observed performances. One of the loudest voices of body language is the hand. The phrases "limp wrist" and "talk to the hand" should make this point clear. Not too surprisingly the foot, especially when bare, is also quite important. Presenting a pointed foot can be quite effeminate.

Attitude is one of the most noticeable of the human characteristics. In our example the man was suave and debonair, the lady coy and bashful. Flip the attitudes and she would be a "hussy" and the man "immature".

Dancing with a masculine attitude will tend to remove the effeminate body language from the performance without any special effort. When you are being "the MAN" all this happens on a subconscious level, effeminate body language just does not fit. That is what the female audience wants to see. You just may find the "Wild Untamed Beast" or the "Romance Novel Hero" in your performance.

The costume, in which you perform, can add a great deal to the impact of your show. It can also totally destroy the image you are trying to project in your performance.

Back to our example, what if the man was wearing the same evening gown as the lady? Male costume cannot be the same as the female costumes without losing impact, or worse. I have seen performances in "unisex" costumes, and while they were excellent shows, a lot of spice was lost by making the male and female dancer look the same. You end up with a not really male, not really female compromise. That for me is the key word "compromise". It means you gave up something that you could have used to fuel the fire of your show. I know it is a very Broadway style of things, but I do have a personal bias, which I am expressing.

Male costume can draw on many sources, from folk-loric to fantasy. Lawrence of Arabia is a good look. If you lean toward Flamenco, Spanish bullfighters had some very impressive looks. Dress uniforms may also be your cup of tea. Male mirror vests from India, especially with harem pants, are another good look. If you are a "Buff" fellow you might consider the Conan look.

A few observations I have made along the way about costuming include:

Costumes that "tease" are effeminate.

V shapes (belts etc.) in the crotch area are for females.

See-through fabrics "tease" and therefore are effeminate.

Short vests and shirts that leave the midriff bare, can work .

Necklines of a masculine cut are crucial for a male look, especially with bare midriffs.

All lines in common with a bra must be missing from torso coverage.

Fringe on a male should not cover bare skin, another "tease".

Costumes framing bare shoulders are for females.

Your complexion and skin colouring limit the colours you should wear; some colours are just feminine.

Less can be more, as in less exposed, less glitzy, less busy.

Whatever your costume, be sure it will survive dancing—intact.

So you are still with me, I guess you are thinking about becoming a Male Belly Dancer?

Here are a few things you should know.

Reasons to give up the whole idea;

>   You don't love the dance form.
>   You don't like people.
>   You don't respect women.
>   You cannot accept women in a leadership role.
>   You are not willing to push your limits, either physically or emotionally.
>   The fact that some male Mid-Eastern dancers are "gay" and dance in a very effeminate style totally gives you the "willies".

Are you still with me? If so here is how to get started:

First and most important learn the Dance. Find a good teacher who will put up with the hassles of teaching a male student, and who, perhaps, is familiar with how he should dance.

Drill the basics. Practice and more Practice.

Lose the extra weight and tone up those muscles. Good warm ups and practice will do this on its own, if done often enough and of sufficient duration.

Put a dance costume together, it need not be elaborate, just appropriate.

If you can, video tape your performances and use them as a tool to develop the stage image you wish to have.

Improve your physical appearance—good posture is very important!

Have close friends critique and help refine your dance.

Go for it, start with small informal venues, and keep dancing.

When you can, go to Mid-Eastern dance workshops and seminars.

Enjoy the dance and follow your heart.

Male dancers are not new to Mid-Eastern dance. Various historical references are made regarding males involved in the dance. True, this is often in a female impersonation role, but other references are to males dancing as males. One of the best-known and most experienced of male Mid-Eastern dancers in the USA, is Bert Balladine. If you ever have a chance to meet him or take a workshop with him, do so, it will be well worth your time.

ANKH

Zaïda—special thanks to Ankh for his invaluable advice......he has been so supportive ever since I first emailed him; and he was the first person to put a Link to my brand new website, on his website. I still cherish the thrill I felt when I saw my Link on his site and his ever so charming comment.

A recent survey conducted in Australia showed that more than 76% of men actually do some form of DANCE, but sometimes only in private. This shows that men have the same innate desire to dance as do women.

My husband, Mike and I have worked up a duet routine which is a bit comic and very light-hearted.

Mike does hand movements involving closed fists and thrusts from the shoulder; I do fluttery, feminine movements to provide a wider contrast.

We have not included veils, as they do not lend themselves to the 'story'.

Audiences find the dance amusing and a 'bit of fun'. . . . . . Zaïda

Some comments from another male dancer—

The veil is perhaps a good example of what can be learned by a man and adapted.

When I started, a veil would have felt awful weird, although at one time I went to a veil workshop. Since that time, I have noticed male veil dancers—one used a VERY large silk veil; another did a 'signature' double veil routine; one does a very vigorous veil routine, where he, at one point, is on a knee position back bend, and rather wild veil figure 8's over his body.

I have seen an advertisement, which shows a male dancer with a veil, and I have performed a single (heavy fabric) circle veil routine at a Halloween Belly dance show (dancer audience). None of these pieces were feminine, but probably were adapted from some earlier female version.

CHAPTER 9

INTERESTING MOVES

Basic Stance: Knees slightly bent; pelvis tilted to tuck the buttocks **under.** This is not a case of sucking in your tummy muscles, but actually straightening the spine at the pelvis.

Warm up: ALWAYS warm up before you dance and warm down afterwards.

As Rudolph Nureyev said,

'*You need to tell your muscles that you are going to use them; and you need to tell them that you are finished*'.

All exercises are repeated 4 times on each side......if you feel PAIN. STOP!

BREATHING: clears the lungs and helps the lymphatic system.

It is very important to breathe down into the abdomen. Your ribs have limited movement and thus do not allow your lungs to fully expand. By breathing into the abdomen, the lower part of your lungs can SPREAD and expel all that stale air.

See Chapter 7 for detailed exercises.

Remember your Pelvic Tilt.

SNAKE ARMS—hold the arms out sideways at shoulder level and rotate the shoulder joint in the cup. This will cause your elbow to be superior or inferior to your arm as you rotate your shoulder and, by letting this movement flow down to your wrists, you will get a snakelike undulation along your arms.

Remember your Pelvic Tilt.

SHIMMY: This is excellent for warming you up on a cold day, or for an aggravation displacement activity if you are delayed in a queue.... may make the person who is causing the delay, hurry up, in case you are about to take a fit!

Stand with both feet slightly apart and drum the heels, alternately on the floor. This will make the muscles in your thighs work. THIS is the feeling you need to focus upon. With practice you will be able to move these thigh muscles without drumming your heels and you have the start of your shimmy.

In time, as your body loosens up, your shimmy will take shape and you will be able to experiment with it and add it to other movements and walks.

The Shoulder shimmy is just a movement of the shoulders backwards and forwards. The faster the movement, the smaller the distance travelled and you will end up with a shimmy.

Remember your Pelvic Tilt.

CORKSCREW— This is a BIG circle with your hips...stick that bum out and then shove your hips forward.

At the same time make a BIG circle with your chest. Stick your charms OUT, then suck them right back.

Combine these two so that when your hips are forward your chest is back, then your hips go back and your chest comes forward.

At the same time, you walk your right foot around your left foot, which remains in the same position, just pivoting with the body.

Reverse and go the other way.

You arms can do what they please.

Remember your Pelvic Tilt.

EGYPTIAN WALK—This is an advanced variation of the Upward Vertical Figure 8. When your foot takes the weight you drop your hip DOWN. Knee bent, hip down; hip out to side; other foot and hip lifts. Repeat opposite side. Smooth this out into a very fast, very small move, using tiny steps to move around. Take care not to become pigeon-toed. A forward hip swerve may be added as you gain confidence.

Remember your Pelvic Tilt.

CAMEL—This step needs considerable flexibility in the spine. Picture a figure eight with your hips going forwards and backwards, together.

From the Basic Stance take a small step forward, pushing with the other foot so that the torso juts forward and upward. As the feet come together, ripple the torso backwards and down. Imagine you have a loose hinge at the waist-line and you are pivoting your hips and chest backwards and forwards on this hinge, until you get an undulation; taking a small step forward with each repetition. This step will also travel sideways/ diagonally.

It may help to imagine you have received a sharp poke in the back and then a sharp poke in the navel.

SIDEWAYS CAMEL—same movement as the Camel but you travel sideways by doing a form of the grapevine step. Very small steps.

GRAPEVINE —this is a traditional Greek dance step, but is used in many other forms of dance. Travelling to the left, the right foot crosses behind the left foot and takes the weight. The left foot steps to the left and takes the weight, the right foot crosses in front of the left foot and takes the weight. The left foot steps to the left and takes the weight.

Variations can include an up and down wavelike motion as you take the steps, or sharp hops. You can also take a step forward and back before continuing to the left. Or you can travel to the right if you prefer.

Hold your veil at arms width, straight across in front of your body with just your eyes showing above the upper edge or swirl your veil in figure eights above your head as you travel. Limited only by your imagination.

Remember your Pelvic Tilt.

HAGALLA—Upper body is calm; all the movement is in the lower section. Very small steps, not more than the length of your foot. From the Basic Stance, R knee is straight, L knee bent (45°). Weight on the R foot. Shift weight to L foot, knee straight and bend R knee, lifting foot and lifting R hip. Imagine you are a puppet and somebody is pulling your R hip upwards with a thread.

Step onto R foot, knee bent, shift weight onto R foot and straighten knee. Bend L knee, lifting foot and L hip. So that as you step onto a foot the hip jerks up and down with a large downward movement.

A variation, is to slide your hips to the right or the left.

Summary: Bend the straight leg and lift it quickly from the hip before stepping onto the foot and bending the knee. Immediately do the same with the other leg. This is a very quick movement and causes your hips to move up, down, backwards and forwards, creating a great deal of movement with your coin belt.

Remember your Pelvic Tilt.

SURAAH—Very small, VERTICAL rib cage circles, bend the spine only a little bit inward (so your upper body profile looks almost like a C), try to make small vertical rib cage circles again.

Straighten the spine and 'slide' the rib cage to the right and do vertical circles, then slide to the left and repeat the small circles.

A variation is to slide the rib cage to the right, 2 small vertical circles, a horizontal half circle across your front, then 2 small vertical circles on the left, then a horizontal half circle across your back.

Remember your Pelvic Tilt.

Zaïda's SHIMMY—Start your shimmy at the hips, let it imperceptibly move up to the chest, then as imperceptibly to the head, then back down again. As the shimmy leaves the hips, the hips become stationary and the movement is all in the chest, then the chest becomes stationary and only the head moves.

This will take a bit of practice to get the isolations and to get the flow of the movement so that it becomes almost an undulation. Very effective and always produces a gasp from the audience.

Remember your Pelvic Tilt.

BELLY RIPPLE—Relax your body. Feet parallel and knees slightly bent, stomach muscles pushed out slightly. Start tilting the pelvis upward, whilst pulling in the stomach muscles. The arch in your back should be nearly straight. Make a 'wave' backward, then forward with your pelvis. Slowly relax your abdominal muscles and bend slightly forward at the waist, creating a 'rippling' movement of back and hips.

> **WARNING:** *this move may cause diarrhoea*
> *if repeated more than a few times each session.*

- Remember your Pelvic Tilt.

PEACOCK WALK—Basic stance…leading with the hip, **slowly** drag one foot around to the front….dragging the top of the toes on the floor. Tentatively tap the ground lightly with the tip of your big toe (as if you were a peacock, disturbing insects in the ground). Place that foot down and repeat move with other foot.

Very small, delicate steps in a straight line as if walking a tightrope…slide, tap, step—slide, tap, step.

Add snake arms, holding a veil—or you can shimmy the veil up high, behind you as if it were the peacock's beautiful tail. Pause after a few steps, bend the front knee and lock the back knee across the calf of the front leg, flutter the snake arms with veil. Rise and repeat sequence.

Remember your Pelvic Tilt.

WASHING MACHINE—Swivel your hips forcefully whilst walking forwards with tiny steps. Keep the upper body still. Picture those old-fashioned washing machine agitators. Warning, may cause diarrhoea if prolonged.

Remember your Pelvic Tilt.

PEEK A BOO!—this is a very intricate step at first, but very simple once you have mastered it (like the Shimmy).

I will do the feet first.... the left foot remains in position and only swivels as you turn to the left. The right foot lunges forwards and then backwards.

Now the arms....... the left hand cups your head next to the left ear, without actually touching your hair. The right hand lunges forward with the right foot, then as that foot lunges backwards the left hand lunges forward and the right hand touches the left cheek with the back of the right hand.

At the same time you tilt your left ear downwards and look backwards over your right shoulder.

This is a very cheeky move if you look straight at someone with slightly lowered eyelids when you point forwards with the right hand lunge and then look slyly at someone else over your right shoulder.

Do two lunges in each direction.... North, West, South, East.

Remember your Pelvic Tilt.

BACKWARD JUMP—small jump to the right, small jump to the left, step forward on right foot, forward on left foot swivelling around in a half circle so that you continue in the same direction as you take two sharp leaps backwards with both feet together, body bent forwards at waist. Push both hands forwards to make the move appear much larger.

This is an attention getter if several dancers all do this in unison and their belts all 'chink, chink' at exactly the same time.

HEAD SLIDES—This isolation moves the head on the neck.... sideways. Left to right. The body and shoulders remain still and the head.... slides. Be sure to keep the head absolutely upright and not tilt the chin to the side.

To get the feel, place your little fingers on your collar bones on either side of your neck, the thumbs are held upright and almost touching your cheeks. Move your head so that your right cheek touches your right thumb, then the other side...to the left. Make sure you do not tilt your chin to make your cheek touch your thumb. As your neck muscles gain flexibility, you will be able to move the thumbs further and further apart until you do not need this prop and can do head slides, *'look Mum, no hands!'*.

Once you have gained sufficient neck movement, hold your hands close to your chest in the 'prayer' position. This creates a centre marker point to emphasise the head movement. You can hold one hand at your chest and one hand above your head, but still in the 'prayer' position even though they are separated by your head and thus form a frame.

You can hold both hands above your head in the 'prayer' position, thus framing your head with your elbows. The ideas are limitless.

An alternative to the head slide is to keep the head immobile and to slide the body.

Keep your head still and slide the entire body to left or right. Make sure you do not counterbalance your hips by leaning your chest the other way.

The whole body must remain upright and as a single shape, maintaining perfect alignment. Totally upright.

VEILS

The aim, when dancing with a veil, is to get as much air UNDER the veil as possible so as to make it FLOAT.

Hold one long hem veil across the front of your body just below shoulder level, with your hands about 12 inches outside the line of your body, on each side.

Grip the edge of the veil between thumb, closest to the body, and the index finger on the outside of the veil. The rest of the fingers are used to PUSH the veil in the direction of travel, thus giving it lift.

FIGURE EIGHT

Drop your right hand, whilst pushing the veil with those fingers, and lift the left hand taking the veil up over your head and down behind you. The right hand follows the left hand in a circle above the head and round the back.

As your hands come to the left behind your head, drop the left hand and the right hand follows it, bringing the veil back to the start position.

This is a basic figure eight and is the centre of almost all veil moves. It is also a very good move when you need a rest.

You can do fast figure eights, or slow ones, turning the body at the same time. They all look like different moves but are all basically the same move.

HIP FLICKS WITH VEIL

Moving sideways to the right, do hip flicks with the right hip.

The veil is held behind you, low down, with the left hand touching the right hip, this gives you a lot of veil to flick.

The right hand flicks the veil slightly behind your line of travel so that as you step you do the hip flick and flick the veil at the same time, but don't step on the veil as you move.

TUMBLING VEILS

Veil is held across the front of the body. Left hand touches right shoulder. Right hand brings veil between veil and body, makes a complete forward and back circle giving the veil a big flick. Reverse the circle, bringing the veil forward in a big flick.

Left hand drops to left side of body. Right hand touches left shoulder. Left hand brings veil between veil and body and makes a complete forward and back circle giving the veil a big flick. Reverse the circle, bringing the veil forward in a big flick.

Get this movement going really fast and it looks absolutely fantastic.

YIPPEE

Hold the veil by the upper hem across the front of the body. Throw the veil straight up and catch the lower hem as you step forward under the veil and let it drop down behind you, but still holding the veil. I call this YIPPEE, because that is what I say when I achieve this without getting smothered in the veil.

A simpler version which makes a striking finale, is to throw the veil up, step forward under it and let the veil drop to the floor behind you.

OOPS!

If you drop your veil in the middle of a dance, pretend it was intentional and make it a part of your dance. If you have only dropped one end, you can step backwards and pull the veil towards you like a snake, until you get control of that pesky critter again.

If you drop the whole shebang, then you need to dance around the veil as if you wanted to do just that and after acting as though you are 'talking' to that veil, you can gracefully dip and grip the nearest portion of its anatomy.

CAMEL

This step lends itself beautifully to holding the veil high above your head in both hands and letting it drape down your back as you do the Camel.

Or you can hold the veil across the front of your body and hold your hands high above your head, but behind the line of body, so that the veil is just below your face and forms a frame.

SENSUAL

Hold the left hand high above the head behind the line of body. The veil is behind the body. The right hand sweeps low across the front of the body while you step to your left and dip low. Rise out of the dip and do a slow and sultry reverse circle with your whole body.

Change hands so that the right hand is high above the head behind the line of body. The left hand sweeps low across the front while you step to your right and dip. Rise up and do the reverse circle. Lovely with slow music.

CHAPTER 10

REPARTEE—1999

*'Age is only important when it comes
to dead fish and good wine'*

Women—and men, have been sending me their comments from many countries:

AUSTRALIA —Brisbane, Qld; Kununnurra, WA; Melbourne, Vic; Sapphire, Qld; Seaforth, Qld; Stanthorpe, Qld; Sydney, NSW.

BELGIUM—

SWEDEN—Stockholm

U. K. —London, England.

U. S. A. —Alaska, Boston, California, Camarillo, Florida, Georgia, Hawaii, Idaho, Minnesota, Oklahoma, Oregon, Sacramento, San Francisco, Texas, Utah.

MUST BE THE BANGLES

'I love your site, and I am fascinated that you come from the coastland of Australia.

I started dancing at the age of 30, in San Francisco, and have done it off and on since.

I have always been BIG, and I am almost 50.

On Halloween, I dressed up in belt and dancing bra and some scarves, for work. I got, let us say, lots of male attention even though I am big. Must be something about the bangles.

I am happy that you are encouraging older women to dance. Please keep up the good work'

Zaïda: Thank you for your very kind words. I am absolutely thrilled to be encouraging older women to learn belly dancing.

WE HAVE LIFT OFF!

'I've just started teaching and really like what you say. Now I know how to encourage any older woman who wants to dance but feels intimidated because she's not 19. Thanks'

Zaïda: This is exactly what I hoped to achieve. There must be THOUSANDS of older women out there who wanted to learn to belly dance, but felt they were too old.

I discovered belly dancing 3 years ago at the age of 60 and my health has progressively improved until now, my husband says I am living proof of the health benefits of belly dancing. I am healthier now, than at any time in the past six decades. Keep shimmying!

LIVE MUSIC

'I've been belly dancing for 23 years, so since I didn't start at birth, I'm not a spring chicken. We have a troupe with members in their 20's, 30's, 40's, and had a dancer in her 50's (she is fabulous).

We have LIVE MUSIC too, which I love.'

Zaïda: Oh! How I ENVY you, your LIVE MUSIC.

I wish we could get some musicians motivated to set up a Middle Eastern Band, here in Mackay.

BEHIND THE VEIL

'I think a lot of young people think silver hair means the brain's gone as well, (I am 59), and I'm sure some of the younger dancers think I'm a bit of a curiosity churning out brochures and flyers and stuff, which silver haired people are not supposed to know about.'

NORTH TO ALASKA!

'Thankyou for letting me know that at 53 and learning to belly dance, I am not the only 'older lady' taking belly dancing up.

Although I am overweight, I find it is the best exercise I can do. I love to dance. This is more fun than stair stepping. It is so graceful and it works all the body.'

Zaïda: Within three years you will feel 35 again. Guaranteed. I will be 64 next year and feel 35. My health has been better, since I started belly dancing, than it ever was for the previous 60 years.

I am so THRILLED to be reaching all the women who WANT to dance, but feel they are too old/heavy.

Dancing will fix both those concerns.

A ROSE BY ANY OTHER NAME . . . .

'What does the name, Zaida, mean?'

Zaïda: The name Zaida means that I have chosen a name which pleases me and which I use as my dancing persona. When I am Zaida I am transported into the world of Oriental Dance and am no longer my ordinary, everyday self.

I strongly recommend that every dancer choose a name which pleases her (or him), and which will transport them into the world of dance, music and sheer enjoyment.

Whether the conjunction of those letters has any specific significance, I have no knowledge, or interest. Presumably some person, some time in the past, has made an arbitrary decision that a particular meaning shall apply to a particular name.

I am **Zaïda!**

I dance! I LOVE it! Choose a name. If it does not feel comfortable…change it. I know one lady who changed her name four times before she found one she really liked. I rather fancied the name 'Sahara'—(as I was born in Africa), when I first started out, but it was too similar to the name of another dancer (here in Mackay at that time), so I chose a different name. I chose **Zaïda**. I added the double dots over the i as this made it different and also indicates that the i is used twice—in the first AND second syllables. Thus Z-EYE-EE-DUH.

(I have since discovered that Zaïda means LUCKY)

HUSBANDS

'My husband is being a bit of a butt head about my dancing. He's not sure he likes me doing this.

A good friend of mine, her husband just flat said "NO!"

I would not go for that. I haven't let a man tell me what to do since I was at home living with my Dad and Mom.

I wish I knew where women get it into their heads that we go from listening to our parents tell us what to do, to listening to our men do it!'

Zaïda: Husbands are missing out on at least 50% of their lives when they do not share their woman's joys and interests. Just as she shares his.

I know a woman whose husband absolutely refused to give her permission to dance in public. So she just danced in class. Eventually she woke up that she did not need his permission. Now she dances every chance she gets; in public; and loves it.

MY husband is my most ardent supporter. He is my PR man, my stage manager, my sound and lighting man and my compere at all my performances.......

Confucius says: *Change what you can change. Accept what you can't change; and learn to tell the difference".*

FEELING the MUSIC

'I found everything you say informative, fun and inspiring.

I am 51. I started dancing in January of this year and am totally committed to it. Your words about the 'feeling' of dancing the music and being relaxed and yourself are so true. I danced in a student show in a restaurant in July and plan to do another performance soon.

You are so right about dancing for friends, especially women. A group of us women, here in Oregon, are doing a river rafting trip next month and I was asked if I would perform for them one of the nights we're camping!

Of course—my FAVOURITE audience is my boyfriend!

You are a true inspiration. I'm glad I found you'.

Zaïda: I receive such an enormous amount of support for my dancing, especially in this IYOP (International Year of the Older Person), that I hope to pass on some of this to other 'older' women. Keep dancing.

Aloha from HAWAII

'At 43 I had my first bellydancing class yesterday! I am not a very athletic person and have 'two left feet'; but I can totally get into this and am anxiously awaiting my next class!

I feel a little self conscious about my size, which is BIG...I have lost 63 lbs and now weigh 227, and am still working hard to lose more...but I am still going to give it my best shot!!! '

Zaïda: Don't feel that BIG is a disadvantage in Belly dancing. You don't have to work as hard. Get that shimmy going and it keeps on keeping on. Skinny bodies have to work much harder.

EXERCISE VIDEO

'Do you have a video for sale with the same instructions that you have here?'

Zaïda: I only do belly dancing for the sheer joy of dance. I do not sell. If I can encourage older women to share my passion, then that is what it is all about. I hope you can find a suitable video somewhere. Sorry I cannot help with your quest.

A NEW BEGINNING

'I live in the U.S.A. in the Midwest and just found a teacher in a city very near me.

Now, I am going to start belly dancing lessons in September. I was really beginning to wonder if I really was nuts, but now am glad to see that I am not alone!

I had been going over the decision in my head (especially after I saw the look on my husband's face…total surprise :: grin::)….wondering if I was just wanting to be someone I am not; but although I am a very quiet person I have been involved in community theatre (my biggest lead was playing 'Truvy' in Steel Magnolias) and dancing.

Something 'turns on' when I am on stage that I cannot explain.

I have raised three boys and have six grandchildren, but still consider myself to be attractive and don't feel anything like everyone seems to say women are supposed to feel at this age. In fact, I think I look better and KNOW I feel better about myself than I did in my 20's.

So let them laugh. You have certainly put the period on the end of my decision.

How long do you think it will take to learn enough to actually be able to dance in front of an audience? I want to learn to do it correctly.

Also, I have heard there is a body stocking that can be worn. I have a nice figure but a terrible surgical scar that goes from the bottom of my chest to the bottom of my tummy and cannot picture in my mind how in the world you could wear a body stocking and look like a belly dancer. In fact, ::grin:: I'm not even sure what a body stocking is!

When I turned 50, (I think my family thought I was nuts)—first, I sent in a resume, interviewed and became a flight attendant for American Airlines.

I was already taking a jazz and tap dance class and was the youngest in my class.

Thank you so much for the encouragement to go ahead with this.'

Zaïda: You have told me that I am achieving exactly what I set out to achieve.... to encourage older women to learn to belly dance.

I have received nothing but support from the people who know me, and I wanted to pass on this encouragement to people who do not live in such a supportive community. Never let other people's hang-ups rule your life. You don't want to live THEIR lives, so don't let them try to live YOURS!!!!!

Don't worry about DOING IT RIGHT! There is no right or wrong. Who is supposed to be the 'boss cocky' who says this is right and this is wrong? NOBODY! You do it YOUR WAY!

Body stockings are IMPOSSIBLE to wear here in the tropics. If you have a figure fault, design a costume which will cover it. One dancer had a horizontal scar, so she had a dagger tattooed over the scar. Your vertical scar can easily be covered with drapes, fringes, beading, anything that works for you. I have an hysterectomy scar, which just peeps out above my skirt. If it bothers anyone—it does not bother ME!

Your husband will be THRILLED with his dancer wife, once he understands what it means in terms of your health, flexibility, self esteem, sheer sensuality.

I have four great-grand-children.......all girls…

INSPIRATION!

'Hello, Zaida: I am a pup at a mere 29 going on 30 but was delighted and inspired by you. I want to thank you and all the other 'elderly women' for being an inspiration to me.

I have just started to learn belly dancing in Minnesota, USA and have loved every class! I find that my time is short for practice outside of class and as I come closer to turning 30 I keep wondering what part of my body will be the next to 'give out' [my first grey hair arrived at 21].

You are all my living proof that I do not even have to consider giving up this glorious passion as I age.

Also, to all belly dancers, thank you for being out there and showing the world the truth [where fashion and Hollywood have failed], in that most women are a size 12 or larger [nothing personal against anyone thinner as we know everyone should be proud of who they are; but the reality just isn't there and it hurts to see young women who will never get to be less than a 12 and try to kill themselves doing it]. I personally am a size 18 and proud of it.

So let's shimmy those HIPS, because that's why we have them!!

Some may consider you 'elderly' but you will always be knowledgeable, graceful, beautiful and inspiring to me. Perhaps in a couple or so decades I'll have the opportunity to pass down your inspiration to others to continue and not give up because of age or fear of getting older.'

Zaïda: I felt very flattered by your comments. My aim is to encourage women not to be intimidated by the fact that they are no longer young, nubile and skinny.

I read somewhere that it is nature's design for older women to become fat, so as to encourage the males of the species to breed with the younger women who would produce more viable offspring. This may be the case—who knows?—but we don't stop being women just because we are older, and we still have the same feelings as we had when younger.

Belly dancing allows us to express those feelings.

I plan to be dancing thirty years from now, so you have about 6 decades ahead of you......hang in there....

DANCING AT THE TOP END

'I lived in Mackay for 12 months and didn't even know you were there. I am now living in the Kimberley in the north of Western Australia.

We have started a small group with a lot of help from an instructor in Perth. So far our group is going well, with about 15 die-hard fans. We have been together as a group or troupe for about 9 months now and have had a small debut performance and one appearance at the local mardi gras, with two of us also dancing at local parties.'

Zaïda: It is a real thrill to hear that belly dancing has reached the Top End of Australia.

We have felt the surge of interest flowing through the continent and this is truly encouraging for the people living in isolated communities.

Australia has no National Dance as such, not like Irish Dancing or Scottish Dancing, so Belly Dancing is taking a real grip on the population. We will take it and mould it to our own psyche and not worry too much about how it is done in other countries. We are just there for the sheer joy of dance.

I MUMBLE "Belly Dance"

'I tend to mumble "belly dance" in answer to questions about what kind of dance classes I'm taking!

At age 47 I felt a little old, but I love the dance and music so much!

My adult children think it's great, and my granddaughter enjoys dancing with me around the living room.

I lack the confidence to dance in public, though.

Someday! By the way, I live in California—U.S.A.'

Zaïda: At 47 you are still a young woman. At 63 I am still a young woman. Some women are old at 29. I can remember feeling really old at that age. Now, chronological age is not a factor in my life. Mental age, and physical well-being are what counts.

If you THINK young, then you ARE young. As one lady said to me, "I don't see myself the way the mirror reflects my image".

I totally agree. In my mind I see myself as 35, the perfect age for a woman…old enough to know what she is doing and young enough to do it.

My grandson of 25, who is also my Webmaster, sends my photograph to all his friends on the Internet and says, "This is my Granny". (He has two daughters……)

When you are ready to perform in public, choose a sympathetic group, like an Aged Persons' Home. They are starved for entertainment, and a very receptive audience.

I have danced at several of the homes here in Mackay, and they are always saying,

"When are you going to dance for us again?".

You see, my husband and I have a musical duo, I play alto sax and sing alto, and he plays electronic accordion, so we visit the Homes and Hostels regularly with our music.

If you enjoy your dance, your audience will enjoy it too. They will be able to fantasise that it is them, up there dancing. Give them their fantasies.......

PERFECT BODIES

'Hi, I teach at two belly dance classes. Although one of my classes has fairly young women (35 to 45), they are not necessarily 'perfect' bodies; (weight 200 to 250lbs = {91—113kgs}).

My point is that being young does not ensure a 'perfect' figure. I suppose they may have been more so, when younger, but they were still too tall, or heavy, even then. So we of course work on all the other important parts of the dance: Costuming; Interesting choreography; Presentation, etc.

For the most part, the women have seemed very accepting over the years, but that may be in part due to my attitude. If I seem to have paid my (dance) dues, and am interested in the dance (not the female dance students), I think that there is pretty good acceptance.

I am careful to be appropriate to my venue and audience.

Also, I read about the male dancer (**Ankh**), and I agree about the styling, and about learning everything, and then discarding or modifying what you don't like. In fact women wind up doing this, as well.

The veil is perhaps a good example of what can be learned by a man and adapted. When I started, a veil would have felt awful weird, although at one time I went to a veil workshop in Idaho. But since that time, I have noticed male veil dancers—one used a VERY large silk veil; another did a 'signature' double veil routine; one does a very vigorous veil routine, where he, at one point, is on a knee position back bend, and a rather wild veil figure 8's over his body; I have seen an ad which shows a male dancer with a veil, and I have performed a single (heavy fabric) circle veil routine at a Halloween Belly dance show (dancer audience). None of these pieces were feminine, but probably were adapted from some earlier female version.'

(A male dancer of 43).

Zaïda: What a lucky little chappy you are—teaching women to belly dance. You must be the envy of everyone you know.

My husband is dead keen to learn to belly dance, but my teacher is reluctant to take on men, in case she attracts the wrong sort; and she does not want to include my husband in her women's class, in case the women drop-out—which is a real problem here in Mackay (rhymes with eye).

So, I am teaching him some of the moves I have learned and he is really enjoying it. I am also making him work with a veil, it certainly requires a bit of muscle power to get that veil moving, and that is far better than pumping iron at the gym—BORING!

MIRACLE

'I really enjoyed your comment: quote— 'The nice people will be happy for you, when they see how much you are enjoying yourself. The others don't exist'

I love it !! I started belly dancing at age 42 and am still dancing 20 years later! I don't look or feel twenty years older and I know the dance has contributed greatly to this miracle. Thank you for a wonderful page. '

Zaïda: We are proving that dance is for EVERYONE, especially belly dance......

MAINTAINING INTEREST

'I'm giving a series of 4 classes to the local weight-loss group, starting tonight, and will tell them about you — (I think they are about 45—I'm nearly 38).

So far I haven't had much success in maintaining long-term interest in belly-dance, but maybe this will be the new beginning???

I held classes for about 6 months last year, but the numbers just dwindled away.

It gets very cold here and people seem to want to hibernate!

I originally learned to dance in Brisbane and moved here 3 years ago. I too suffer from the isolation problem and really wish I could find some women here to share my passion for MED (Middle Eastern Dance). Women always say to me they would love to learn, but when it comes to the crunch they back out. I just have to keep trying.'

Zaïda: We also have a very high drop-out rate here, in Mackay. A few suggestions, which come to mind—perhaps you could set up a daytime dance and coffee session, so that it is more of a social than a class. You could also do a few demonstration dances at places like old folks' homes. They are a very appreciative audience and talk to their rellies about the entertainment, which comes to them. The more people who hear about belly dance, the more students you are likely to attract.

Also, dancing in public gets the adrenalin flowing and those who are brave enough to join in will say, "When's the next one?".

I wish you luck in attracting at least a few enthusiastic dancers.

FAST SHIMMY

'I found it was encouraging to know there are so many other older dancers out there.

I danced in my twenties, left it in my thirties, and am returning to it in my late forties; but one of the frustrating things for me is that I can no longer shimmy (fast, that is).

I could shimmy really fast when I was in my twenties, but although I've stayed with it and practiced for over two years now, I just can't shimmy fast anymore; its discouraging. Any hints?'

Zaïda: Welcome to the fraternity of belly dancers. It is lovely having contact with dancers from all over the world.

I feel that shimmying (is there such a word?) is a matter of being relaxed. The more uptight you become the less you are able to shimmy. Don't work at it, just let it happen.

Beginners work too hard at shimmies, especially shoulder shimmies and their movements are too large. I was helping a new dancer the other day, and when she made her movements very tiny and relaxed her shoulders, she was able to get the embryo of a shimmy going. With practice she will conquer this movement.

I feel that your problem is that you KNOW you used to be able to shimmy 'real fast' and when it did not come back easily, you tensed up. I hope this is a helpful suggestion? Keep dancing.

SELF CONFIDENCE

'At 46, I sometimes feel I'm crazy wanting to use it (belly dancing) for anything but exercise. I started about 10 years ago and have been doing it off and on. There are a few dancers my age that I'm starting to find out about, but usually I'm surrounded by new age youngsters from the colleges. Partly because of lack of self confidence, I've yet to choose a dance name.'

Zaïda: I must admit, that if my first teacher had not been 72, I would never have pursued belly dancing. Now, it is an absolute PASSION. I am in great demand, dancing for older groups of people. I think they all feel envious and wish they had the courage to try something like this, themselves. A mature woman can bring much more to the dance than youngsters. You can express your maturity and joy of BEING. You can express sensuality. Physical appearance is not the same as charisma. Have fun, and choose a dance name SOON. It will give you a new identity and take you out of your everyday life. When I become Zaïda, I am WOMAN.

DANCING IN PUBLIC

'I don't want to dance in public. I don't want the people at work to know I am doing this'

Zaïda: There is no pressure to dance in public, until you are ready. You will find, as your confidence and your ability increase, that just dancing in a class situation will no longer please you. Like a fledgling, you will be ready to FLY. Once you have experienced that surge of adrenalin, which you get from dancing for an audience, you will be asking, 'When's the next one?'.

I am sure the people at your place of work will be happy for you and you may be surprised to find that they start inviting you to dance at functions they are organising privately. Live your life for yourself. You are not hurting anyone by dancing—just the opposite, you will bring joy to other people's lives. Wait until you are ready, then enjoy yourself.

ACHES AND PAINS

'I'm 35, so I really don't consider myself an older woman yet, but I think belly dance is fantastic since it is a dance we can do for our whole life!

As I've gotten older I've noticed that if I don't dance I feel a lot stiffer and have more aches and pains! Belly dance is also great for your posture and upper body strength!

Did you mention beledi dresses in your costuming section? They are sexy, authentic, and keep one covered up! They have always been my preferred style, even when I was 21 and didn't have much to hide! Also, there are patterns available for great ghawazee and Turkish coats that are soooo cool!

Any way, great job and happy dancing!!!'

Zaïda: Before I started belly dancing I had reached the stage where I had to hold onto the railings when descending stairs. Now I can trip down stairs without much thought. So not only your upper body gains strength.

Costuming is a very personal decision and each dancer must suit her personality and preferences. Here, in Mackay, we are in a tropical zone with very high humidity. So less is better when we are dancing. We usually end up damp from head to foot so costumes need to be washable.

Patterns are almost non-existent so we copy from other dancer's costumes and modify to suit ourselves.

HEALTH, ATTITUDE AND COSTUMING

'You have a lot of good information on the health benefits of belly dancing that I was not aware of. I found your tips on costuming very helpful and the section on attitude was so perfectly written.

I started taking belly dance lessons for fun and relaxation thinking I would probably quit after I saw all the young perfect bodies in class. I was happy to find out that there is so much more to this dance than having a perfect physique. I have learned a lot in the year and a half I have been taking lessons and have enjoyed every minute of it

P.S. I wanted to ask you where you got your tassel belt. I have not seen one like it.'

Zaïda: Re the tassel belt—it started out as a very basic coin belt. I added the tassels, then some big coins, then, a second coin belt over the original belt—I took it off its chain and clipped each dangly section to my base belt. The second belt is lightweight, jangly things and very shiny gold—it shimmies at the lightest move. The belt is getting heavier and heavier. It may collapse some day ::Heh! Heh!::

The tassels are just gold tassels from a shop, which sells sewing notions. I think they are meant as Xmas decorations. I have also added some gold strings of beads on each hip. These flounce delightfully. They are definitely Xmas decorations and much stronger than I anticipated. They put up with two classes a week as well as performances. I have just done my 14th performance (in public, I mean) and feel happier and happier about my dancing.

Go for it! The audience can pick up your enjoyment and this lifts them and takes them flying with you.

ENCOURAGEMENT

'I am Spanish, and dance Raqs Sharqi since 1993, when I was 50.

By chance I found you and I felt so well after reading you.

I have always been dancing with younger people and maybe because of that it took me longer to learn, and probably because my back, my bones and my ears—to understand everything is said—showed my age. And truly, I have never been encouraged in my classes or workshops.

However, I never gave it up. I worked hard and enjoyed a lot doing so…

My remaining problems is my balance; I find a little bit difficult to turn, but I try once and again….

Thank you for encouraging older people. I needed it!'

Zaïda: I have also had problems with balance and spins, but I practice a little each day and my balance is improving noticeably. I can now stand on tiptoe for quite a while and I am getting more and more agile in the spins. Keep working at it, a little each day.

NEVER, NEVER think that younger, slimmer dancers are BETTER. They are DIFFERENT. Everybody interprets the music in their own way and that is what makes bellydancing so special. You don't HAVE to try and do it one way, like in ballet.

You are the only dancer in the WORLD who can dance the way you do. You are SPECIAL. Enjoy yourself. I have never had so much fun as I am having now, and I will be 63 on 31st July, 1999.

ISOLATION

'I am one of ten members of a bellydance group in a small town in Central Queensland, Australia. We started in March 1998 with Michelle as our teacher. Michelle has left the area two months ago to work in Brisbane, and now we are 'teacherless'.

I try to gather info from everywhere to study and show the other ladies what I have learnt, every Thursday. We hire a hall, with help from our local Multi-purpose Centre. I happen to be the Admin. Assistant there, which makes it easier. We are trying to receive a grant from the Government, but that's a bit tricky.

Last year, we had a visit in Emerald from Rasheeda and she taught us a lot with her workshop, but we need more, more, more. Could you give us a kickstart, on where to order CD's and Instructional video's etc? Everything seems to be in America. Thanks'.

Zaïda: It is fantastic that you have started a group in a town with a population of less than 600. Please give all the girls my heartiest welcome. Tell them the thing I have learnt, which has the most value to me, is that flexibility is mental, more than physical. If they can overcome their hangups they will find their bodies become fluid, like oil.

Rasheeda did a workshop for us here in Mackay and it was very energising being in a group of women who were all interested in bellydance.

Zaïda

CHAPTER 11

REPARTEE—2000

'Age is only important,
when it comes to dead fish and good wine'

Women—and men, have been sending me their comments from many countries—see Repartee 1999.

New countries 'writing' in 2000....

AUSTRALIA—New South Wales;

AUSTRIA—

CANADA—Nova Scotia; Victoria BC;

DENMARK—

ITALY—

UK—London; Liverpool;

U.S.A.—Florida; Maine; Maryland; Massachusetts; New York City; Northern NY; Oregon; Philadelphia; Seattle; Southern California; Texas; Virginia; Weed, CA;

DO NOT!

'I would just like to say that your messages concerning belly dance are also conducive to younger women.

I have only recently 'discovered' this wonderful art; but the 'DO NOT's' you mention are also embedded in my generation's psyche. After all, my Mom matured in your generation and carried those lessons to me.

My daughters also are learning and discovering this beautiful, ancient art and I absolutely LOVE watching them on their road to self-discovery and maturity.

Thank you for an excellent reference site!'

Zaïda: Self-discovery is what it is all about and not living our lives by someone else's hang-ups. You don't have to be super-wonderful or have a perfect technique. Just ENJOY!

AT HOME!

'I really felt 'at home' reading through your homepage. I found, also, the explanation of some techniques by Botticelli very useful.

When I watched the videos I felt as if I were in a dance class and not in my university. I would have preferred to be in that class!

I was very lucky to find a book by the German dancer, Dietlinde Karkutli. I love her book and every time I open it I see something (the description of a movement or important advice) that I didn't seem to have noticed before. It is really sad that she died some years ago; but I still feel the energy that comes out of her words, as if she were alive.

There is a picture of Dietlinde showing the right position to stand (knees flexed, shoulders back). I learned to keep this position and could feel the incredible reactivation of my belly muscles!'

Zaïda: I am so THRILLED that you have learned the sheer JOY of just letting the music speak to you, instead of dancing someone else's interpretation of the music. I agree that you need to learn the moves, but to DANCE…that is something else.

The knees flexed and shoulders back is part of the stance, but you also need to TILT your pelvis. This is not a matter of sucking in your belly muscles; it is a case of actually tilting the pelvic bones so that your spine straightens out. This takes practice, but if you do this everytime you think about it, you will soon find that it is very uncomfortable to stand in the slouch, which most people adopt. You also need to remain RELAXED.

Easier said than done. But the shimmy only works if your body is as floppy as a jelly.

A REAL GENTLEMAN

'I think that it is wonderful, encouraging women to do belly dancing. It is good exercise. I love watching women do it. I think that belly dancing encourages women to be proud of their bodies and show them off.
Where I am, Middle Eastern restaurants have these shows, and they are very entertaining.
I enjoyed looking at your pictures on your website; it is a very well done site. You are an attractive woman.'

Zaïda: It is truly thrilling to receive a man's point of view on this subject; which is my passion.

ENTHUSIASTIC HUSBAND

'I started belly dancing last year, at age 51. I haven't had such fun in years, and am now taking 2 classes.

I was more than a little horrified when my first teacher more or less insisted that we dance this Summer at all the little local festivals, as I really didn't feel 'good' enough to dance in public. Nonetheless I had a wonderful time and hope to have a solo put together for next Summer.

My husband, a little to my surprise, has been enthusiastic and very helpful; he turned up at all our events with a camera, and video taped the last one. I would probably dance without his enthusiasm, but it's twice the fun if he's having fun too.

My original motivation had much to do with having discovered a great workout, which was really low impact. That shortly gave way to an obsession with the music, the dance and the costume (let's not forget the amusement of the costume), and even had I not lost 5 pounds (only 55 to go), I would have to continue.'

Zaïda: I could not have put it better.

CONSIDERING

'I'm considering trying to do this at 54.'

Zaïda: At 54 you are a whole decade younger than me…. you are still a chicken. GO FOR IT! You will never regret learning belly dancing. You will feel vibrant, healthy, full of life and best of all you will find the hidden YOU! The person who has been suppressed all these years by the admonitions not to 'show off'.

NOW you can dress up with all that 1950's jewellery and put on all the eye make up you can fit onto your face and wear the brightest, sparkliest dresses. You can put glitter in your hair and on your body. You can do what pleases you. That is what belly dancing is all about. Self expression. If you prefer slinky and mysterious, that is just fine. If you prefer loud and exuberant, that is just fine. ENJOY!

Don't hesitate. You will never look back. Open that door and find a whole new world.

AWESOME

'I think your information is Awesome. I have told a young friend of mine—who needs exercise but cannot handle high impact aerobics.

I appreciate your page on Attitude. I think this is a form of exercise that nurtures one's femininity; something that sweating with the oldies just will not do; and it could come in handy for inter-personal entertainment.'

Zaïda: Belly dancing is for EVERYONE. It is as gentle or as vigorous as you like to make it…and you don't have to keep up with anyone else. Also, it makes you feel good about yourself; AND you have a Party Piece.

OLDER—not Oldest

'I danced professionally in the 60's & 70's until I was 42 in 1980. Now I am 62 and 'looking good'. I still have one of the skirts I made in 1965, it will not go round my hips.... about a 6 inch gap.

If I had the nerve, I'd still dance, even if it was for variety, and just to show off. Of course, I guess I fear ridicule, mostly from persons I know; but if I get up the guts, I will do it. After all, I used to teach belly dancing as well.

I feel I am the same person. I don't have a panic attack while dancing.

What was your age when you began, or is it recent? I really envy your courage.'

Zaïda: *Older, not Oldest is the term for us mature dancers. Like wine, we improve with age. Older dancers can bring a 'joie de vivre' to the dance, which younger dancers have yet to learn. We have the poise, the self-confidence, the sensuality, which younger women are still discovering.*

You can make all the moves, but if the inner person is still un-ripe, the flavour will not be full-bodied and I mean that in every sense of the word. Belly dancing is for the full figured woman, who has the right build for the SHIMMY.

I started dancing at the age of 60, four years ago, and have just completed my 40th public performance in those four years. There is a demand out there for the older dancer. Nursing home residents are a very receptive audience. They love entertainment, and many of them have never seen a live belly dancer. I like to 'play up' to the old men. It gives them such a boost. The staff watch apprehensively for signs of a heart attack, but the look of sheer glee on the old gent's face is ample reward.

I never let other people's minds control my life. As long as I am not hurting anyone, I do what pleases ME. Do not allow other people's weird attitudes to life force you into a self-imposed prison. Why should the young people have all the fun? This is our PLAY TIME. ENJOY!

ONLY FOR 'BAD GIRLS'

'I'm 40, have always wanted to belly-dance, but thought it only for 'bad girls'…. that upbringing thing, again.
No classes near me…. can you recommend a good video?'
Zaïda: *Hollywood has a lot to answer for…. belly dance only gained its unsavoury reputation when the word Baladi (meaning music to be accompanied by dance) was mistaken for Belly, as it is pronounced Beh Leh Dee.*

The focus is on the abdominal region, as that is where most female 'problems' occur. Belly dance, over the centuries has evolved to help alleviate 'women's troubles', such as difficult childbirth/menstruation etc. Learning to control and to build the strength in the muscles, thus massaging the internal organs in this area, solves many ills encountered by women, no matter what their age.

I neither teach, nor sell anything, but you may like to look at my Links page at The Art of Middle Eastern Dance. **Shira** has an extremely informative site.

ENCOURAGEMENT

'I'm 56 years old and terribly out of shape; and just starting belly-dancing classes. I'm in such bad shape that I am grateful my teacher is willing to come to my home; I don't think I could handle the train trip, then the class, then the train trip home, with all kinds of subway stairs involved.

However, yesterday I had to walk up many, many flights of stairs because the escalators were broken and I felt an increase in strength in my legs. Can you believe that? After only two classes? This means the class is already helping me.

I think, in a week or two I may be able to take a regular class. I had to sit down for a few minutes during my second lesson, but played my doumbek during that time.

It is really good, if a bit painful, so I think it will only get better after a few classes. She is wonderful and working at my pace entirely. I was the one pushing a bit, since I don't really know my limits at this point.

Thanks for the encouragement and the thoughtfulness, along with all the information. Good work!'

Zaïda: I am so glad you have taken the first steps into the world of belly dancing. I urge you to join a group as soon as you feel sufficiently confident. The sheer energy you get from a group of women all doing something they are passionate about…. you just cannot BUY that; and until you experience it, you will not know what I am talking about.

Belly dancing is not an exercise routine…. although it is about the best form of exercise you may encounter.

Belly dancing is a philosophy for LIFE. Belly dancing will enhance or change your self-image and empower you to be YOURSELF. You will gain self-confidence, poise, inner balance and the sheer joy of living.

As soon as you feel ready, ask your teacher to include you in a group outing with other students in her 'stable'; when they go to an Arabic hafla or restaurant or whatever. You will gain a whole circle of new friends and discover a world you never knew existed.

Of course there are egos, but you learn to flow around them and just ENJOY the essence of the dance. The greatest benefit will be your feeling of well-being as your health and stamina improve.

WEDDING ENTERTAINMENT

'Two of us have been asked to dance at a friend's wedding, whilst the photos are being taken. How do you judge a routine for that type of audience? How do you get the crowd with you?'

Zaïda: My SUGGESTION, and it is only a suggestion…is for you to consider how long the photo session will take, the type of people in the audience and your own preferences.

I would suggest a duet to start; something slinky with veils, and very short, as an introduction and to warm up the audience.

Then you each do a solo to the sort of music you each prefer and can interpret in your own way.

Finally, a duet where you can encourage members of the audience to join in; this would enable you to stretch out the entertainment until the wedding party returns. I suggest you have an encore tune ready in case you need to fill in more time.

If you have a 'lookout' posted to warn you when the wedding party returns you may form a guard of honour by stretching a long veil across the door and keeping it aloft with gentle flits as the wedding party walks underneath.

DISCOVERY

'I found you one day and from that point on, my life has been changed. I am a belly dancer now, due to your insight and encouragement.'

Zaïda: My aim is to tell all women, everywhere about the sheer JOY of bellydance. ENJOY!

CHOREOGRAPHY

'I am a 53 year old belly dancer and I recently moved into a phase of doing little choreography in some solo numbers, particularly if they are done to Arabic 'pop' music.

Recently, a comment from a fellow dancer was repeated to me,

"Oh, you don't choreograph your numbers, you just look as if you are enjoying yourself…and you sing along".

Do I mend my ways, does it really matter?

After all, I do hope to entertain, as well as enjoy myself.

My teachers give conflicting opinions, so I'm asking for an impartial comment from you as you seem to impart a lot of sense.'

Zaïda: You need to understand that many teachers come from a classical ballet background. They have been through years and years and years of rigid training, so they are now brain-wired into dancing to a strict choreography. I think that many of them would find it impossible to dance without a 'script'.

You are not constricted by this indoctrination and can therefore let the music talk to you.

Dancers in Egypt sing along and interact with the audience, and so their dance changes with each audience.

This dance is about having FUN. Do it YOUR way.

One comment I would like to make—if you make eye contact with a male in the audience and his lady is with him—the instant his eyes 'flick', move away. You don't want to embarrass anyone or cause the poor bloke to 'cop any agro' from his lady.

ASTHMATIC

'I have been bellydancing for just over a year now; it was recommended to build lung capacity, as I am an asthmatic with a bum hip.

At first I felt like a klutz, as I am close enough to sixty to be worried and the next oldest person in my class is 30; but I can keep up with them and I have a blast.

A lot of beginners drop out as they have unrealistic goals, like losing 25lbs in ten weeks, without dieting. Those of us who are willing to put in the work, learn a lot, laugh a lot and generally have fun.

You seem to have found that breaking the rules of polite behaviour, which we had drilled into us as girls, as much fun as I do.

We all gain self-confidence, and one of the teenagers, described as shyer than a mouse by her Mum, had the courage to dance in her high school talent show. We all went to support them. They did a fully professional job and, as we noted, were more modestly dressed than many of the girls in the audience!.'

DELI PLUS

'I dance twice a month at a Middle Eastern Restaurant, called Deli Plus in Va. Beach Virginia.'

Zaïda: Good food and bellydancing. HEAVEN!!!!!

TV STAR

'I am 54, and many years ago I belly danced in Germany. I was featured on TV in Baden-Baden for the history of musical instruments.

I don't do the dance now, for one thing, I am totally out of shape and way overweight, but I still love the dance.'

Zaïda: How thrilling to actually be featured on TV.

My aim is to encourage older women to enjoy belly dancing and forget their shape, weight, lack of muscle-tone, colour of their eyes or whatever other reason they can think of to prevent themselves from experiencing the most wonderful thing an older woman can do to keep her body fit and healthy.

As you have danced before, you are WAY ahead of the game and only need the courage to start dancing.

You don't have to wear a cabaret costume, just try the moves and each day you will regain some of your flexibility. ENJOY!

SILK VEILS

'I'm a beginner dancer. I have actually visited Mackay—my grandpa and I went to Queensland in 1994, before the bellydance wave hit! I'll never forget the Rainbow Lorikeets.

Do you know of any sources to order silk veils, online?'

Zaïda: I find that Veils are a very personal choice. It depends on your style of dance. If you want floaty, mysterious, drifting movements, then Silk is the obvious choice. If you want to use a mixture of float and sharp movements, then chiffon has more body.

My personal preference is Crystal Organza, which is fairly stiff and won't drape on your body, but it floats beautifully and has a lot of SNAP for fast movements.

You pays your money and makes your choice.

I am so pleased you have pleasant memories of your stay in Mackay. We get Rainbow Lorikeets infesting a tree in the front of our house whenever the blossoms are in bloom. They all talk at once, at the tops of their voices.

BULGING DISK

'I am now 43, have been belly dancing for about 10 years, and have no intention of stopping for a long time yet!

What I would really like to see is any articles, supporting the health benefit of this dance form.

I am presently recovering from a lower back injury (bulging disk), and would like to be able to show something to my doctor (who knows nothing about belly dancing). I am also planning to see a rehab personal trainer, and would like to get her opinion also.

Any help would be appreciated.'

Zaïda: My information is only hearsay, from professional people, but hearsay all the same. I cannot quote chapter and verse from scientific studies. The proof is in the pudding. I am enjoying better health now, at 63 than I ever did in the past 6 decades.

Strengthening the abdominal muscles will take the strain off your spine. Learning the correct stance will take the strain off your spine. Gaining self-esteem will eliminate stress and thus take the strain off your spine. You would be surprised how much strain on the spine (and internal organs) is generated by stress.

COSTUME GODDESS

'I suppose I qualify as an 'older woman' considering I never took a dancing class 'til I was 40, and that was seven years ago.

I liked the advice you gave to the woman who was self-conscious about her belly. It was almost identical to the advice I give women asking the same question of me.'

BEAUTY GUIDE

'I never thought of it earlier, but I think this could be a great form of exercise and you have so much to offer.

Actually, I am thinking about trying this out! The inches that must come off the waist area must be incredible.'

Zaïda: I am thrilled that you have discovered the value of bellydancing for health. I cannot SHOUT it loud enough. You will feel marvellous within three months and your self-image will be enhanced. Also, you will have a party piece, which will blow the socks off the others doing their soprano songs or gum leaf tunes.

You may not lose WEIGHT, as muscle is heavier than fat, but you will become lean, trim, fit and healthy.

WELLNESS SURVEY

'I am a grad student in Occupational Therapy, writing my pro paper on the therapeutic value of ME dance. I would like any input, feedback, anything at all.

It has been very difficult finding legitimate and credible resources on this subject.

My goal is to contribute to the existing body of knowledge on this subject and make it available to people and practitioners interested in holistic, lifelong wellness.

The wonder of it is, Middle Eastern Dance has so MANY wellness benefits.

The primary focus of my research (a lit review) is mainly to illustrate the natural health-giving functions of ME dance as a daily occupation performed by women (and men).

My question for health practitioners today is, 'if this dance has contributed to the TOTAL well-being of women for so many centuries, could it not still have therapeutic value today?"

VEIL MOVES

'I am an older woman who has just started dancing.

I have learned some incredible veil moves, thanks to you!

I showed my teacher the move I learned from you and she was so excited. It's so nice to be able to give her something back.

Thanks for a great contribution to us older girls You Inspire! Thanks again from the U.S.!!!!!!!!!'

FROZEN TUNDRA

'Your site is an inspiration! It is very refreshing and full of true dance, joy and spirit.

I live in the currently frozen tundra near the Canadian border and have studied, performed and loved Middle Eastern and Mediterranean dance most of my life.

It is a blessed and unique bond of those of us who respond to the hypnotic, elegant, mysterious, joyful sounds of Belly dance music.

I have witnessed so many women over the years who reclaimed a lost part of themselves; or discovered a self they did not realise existed—by the simple act of being involved in bellydancing.

People remark on my youthful appearance and demeanour—though at 50 I know I'm still a spring chicken! I definitely attribute this to my association with Bellydance. This has given me the way to view myself in the world as a passionate and lively woman who grows into age with ripeness. eager for each new adventure. All the many facets of the movements undulations, muscle strengthening hip drops, pops, locks etc. and the yoga-like warmups lead to such a supple body. You just can't beat the benefits.

Many women start this dance at an age when many folks think they can't 'learn new tricks'. But they persevere and blossom. It is the greatest gift.'

QUARTER CENTURY IN THE WINGS

'I took a brief (3 month) Middle Eastern Dance class in Florida, about 25 years and 50 pounds, ago. Recently, I started ME dancing (Middle Eastern), in my 60th year of life, with some nervousness about what the younger classmates would think about it. They and the instructor have been very encouraging.

I also started Feldenkrais bodywork; I believe the combination has given me a healthier body. Quite a treat as I age! Perhaps gracefully.'

Zaïda: You will find your health, your self-image, your joy of living, all enhanced as you progress with your dancing. You will be the envy of much younger people, and you will have a 'party piece' to show off your new skills, once you have gained confidence.

I have received nothing but encouragement from everyone, and am really passionate about belly dancing and its benefits. ENJOY!

JELLY BELLY

'My wife is one of the over 40 gang, and is taking up belly dancing. She feels, as she puts it, a little uncomfortable showing her jelly belly and large belly button.

Her friends tell her that the belly button is the focal point and an important part of the body in order to do 'real' belly dancing. They say that unless you expose your full belly, even well below the belly button, that all your movements will be hidden.

So, what do you think? Is the belly button and belly vital for the dance and necessary to be shown?

My wife awaits your reply. Thanks.'

Zaïda: Please tell your lovely lady that there is no UNIFORM for belly dancing, and one of the most common garments worn is the beledi dress.

This is a straight dress, with slits up the sides. The dress may be made of see-through material, in which case you wear harem pants underneath; or the dress may be made of solid material, in which case your underwear is your own business.

I bet your wife has beautiful ankles, or shoulders, or eyes. Her costume should emphasize her good points and minimize her weaker points.

The modern cabaret costume has been glamorised by Hollywood. I like the cabaret costume, myself, only because I have a terrific waistline for a bird of 63 ::smile::. When I find I feel uncomfortable in a cabaret costume, I will wear a beledi dress. They are lovely.

Belly is a corruption of baladi (pronounced beh-leh-dee) and through common usage in Australia is it now spelled beledi, which means folk dance, or dance of the people, or music to be accompanied by dance.

The absolute essence of belly dancing is to feel comfortable and happy with your own body. You wear the style of costume which makes you feel most comfortable.

In Egypt it is illegal to display the belly button and this must be covered with at least a body stocking. It is considered disgusting to place a jewel in the navel.

The belt is the focus of belly dancing. This, worn low on the hips, will display all your movements, if the belt is designed with lots of dangly, glittery, jingly bits. The weight of the belt 'grounds' your dance and draws attention to the movement of the **HIPS.**

This dance is for sheer pleasure. The fact that it will improve your health beyond your wildest dreams is a major bonus. ENJOY!

Zaïda

CHAPTER 12

REPARTEE—2001

'Few things, which are so good for you,
are also this much fun'.

Women and men have found this Site interesting, and have been sending me their comments from many countries—see Repartee 1999 and 2000.

New countries 'writing' in 2001....

AUSTRALIA: Perth;

ENGLAND: London;

FRANCE:

ISRAEL:

SOUTH AFRICA:

UNKNOWN:

U.S.A: Alaska; Chicago; Ft. Lauderdale; Minnesota; New York; Oklahoma; San Gabriel; Sunnyvale; Tempe; Texas; Virginia; Washington;

FETISH

'My fetish is to be bathed in a belly dancer's body. Neil'

Zaïda: Neil, you can easily achieve this by becoming a belly dancer. Ask at your nearest studio and see if they will accept you as a student. You will need to act like a gentleman.

TOO OLD AT 55!

'Thank you so much for having this site as I thought I was too old (55).

I am an older woman who just took a belldyancing class. The young girl went so fast that I cannot remember many of the moves to practice. I started looking on the Net for some instructions and ran into your site. Where can I go to download some videos?

Zaïda: If you go to my DANCING page and click on aladdin's lamp, you will be taken to Botticelli's site in Denmark. She has some good explanations—with tiny videos—of various hip movements.

If you are in a country which uses PAL video format, go to my LINKS page and look at Yasmin Asar's website…. Yasmin has an excellent teaching video.

If you are in a country which uses NTSC video format, go to my LINKS page and look at the Art of Middle Eastern Dance…. Shira has a plethora of information on her site.

LIGHT INTO THE TUNNEL

'I must tell you that I really enjoyed reading your website. It's almost like a feeling of bringing the light into the tunnel.

I live in Israel and want to study bellydancing but, ironically although living in the Middle East, I can't seem to locate a teacher. Do you have any suggestions?'

Zaïda: You are the first person to speak to me from Israel. WELCOME!

Many women have contacted me about the problem of finding a teacher. I suggest you find a small group of like-minded women and each of you buy a teaching video. Then each of you can bring to the 'class' a move you have learned from your video and teach the others, that way you can correct any 'errors' and learn and ENJOY.

REMEMBER there is no right or wrong way to dance. Listen to the music. Listen to your soul. Learn a few basic moves and have FUN.

Remember also, that belly dance is the dance of the people...it is what people did when music moved them to dance. They did not have formal lessons.

REMOTE AREA

'Dear wonderful role model. I am so thankful for your encouragement for this sensuous dance form. I am most interested but find living in a remote area there are no teachers. What videos/music should I spend my money on? How can I teach myself and not make mistakes?

I am 49 years of age. I want to be devoted but need an instructor I feel. Am I doomed to not be able to learn correctly? I do not want to just mimic movements. I want this very much but just need direction.'

Zaïda: Belly dancing is not a solitary pastime. You need company. You need energy feedback. You need to ENJOY!

Your best bet is to find a group of like-minded women, if there are no classes near you, and form your own group. If you each learn from watching videos, you can help each other to master the moves. The joy of belly dancing is being with other dancers...male and female.

I cannot advise on suitable teaching videos as I have only seen two myself and so am not in a position to judge.

Music is a very personal choice. MY preference is for Westernised, Middle Eastern music where the high pitched, wailing sounds have been avoided. Therefore, I tend to favour Emad Sayyah's music, but unfortunately about 50% of the tunes on any given CD are vocals, so that limits my choice. I only use non-vocals, as I have no idea what they are singing about.

The best thing about belly dance is that it is YOUR dance and there is no right or wrong way to dance. Let the music 'speak' to you. Learn a few basic moves and work on them and you will find yourself inventing your own moves. Each dancer's body moves differently, so even though two dancers may practice the same move, they will look totally dissimilar when they actually dance. (I am not talking about ballet, where the dancers all have to be clones…. Same build. Same height).

GO for it! Ignore other people's opinions. Listen to your SOUL.

QUICK STUDY

'I have a question…. I am a licensed massage therapist and fitness instructor. I am in good shape and am wondering if I could be accepted as a performer belly dancer, (after getting lessons of course). I am a quick study. I am 41 years old.'

Zaïda: As you are already very fit, you would find you are ready to perform after a series of lessons (you will know when you feel ready).

Belly dancing looks very simple, but you will discover a whole world of wonder at just how difficult some of the moves actually are and how much there is to learn. It is a never-ending learning curve.

Your age has no bearing on the subject. I started at 60 and most of my dancers are in their 60's. We perform regularly at the Aged Persons Homes in the area.

TERROR

'In the light of the recent events (the September Eleven attack on the World Trade Centre in New York, and other places), I am so happy to see sites like yours!

As a Muslim who has been under direct back-lash, it is both refreshing and encouraging to see your attitude.

I am so happy to see that not everybody has decided that all Muslims are evil. I am also very pleased to see you encouraging your dancers to be the same.

Keep dancing!'

Zaïda: I am heartsore at the trouble this event has caused throughout the world.

You drop a rock in a pond and the ripples spread FOREVER.

I wrote this letter to my local paper, it was printed this morning. You may find it consoling.

'I had the privilege of meeting Imam Barry Hassan during the preparations for the Barrio Festival held at Caneland Sound Shell in August 1999.

Barry is a true leader, firm but fair; he is a gentleman.

I can relate to the fears of the local Islamic community, as, in Rhodesia during the Second World War, my mother was the target of hatred, as her mother and father, both born in South Africa of Dutch and Austrian parents respectively, marked my mother as a Nazi in the eyes of the community.

My father was British to the core.

I ask the Mackay Community to close ranks and protect our Islamic community from such petty hatred. Our way of life is the envy of Australia and the World, and we must protect our own.'

I hope this nonsense will settle very rapidly. How can anybody hold innocent people responsible for the blind hatred of a very, very small group of sub-humans?

My warmest wishes to you.

OPEN ATTITUDE

'Thank your for your wonderful website. I can sense by the openness of your site that you are a very warm, generous, free spirited Earthmother.

I am your age and I just started taking belly dancing a month ago, and believe me I had every intention of giving it up, this second month, when fees for the class are due.

I am not having a physical problem; I have been an avid walker for 15 years (daily, never missing) and I have been doing various martial arts for 7 years. I am extremely grateful that I am in such good physical condition.

THE PROBLEM was mental. I frankly just felt too mature to start out on such a sensually shrouded form of exercise. I felt much inspiration reading your website, and I think I can continue with the lessons now, with more of an open attitude.

THANK YOU LOVE.'

Zaïda: This is exactly the reason I set up my website. You have truly gladdened my heart. I teach a small group of older women, and they all say how healthy they feel since they have been belly dancing and how much their attitudes to life have changed.

They are so enthusiastic it is sheer JOY to share my limited knowledge of belly dancing with them.

COLD FEET

'I am enjoying bellydance, however, the only cloud is with my feet.... I have a tendency to get a very painful cramping of my two smaller toes in one foot at the most inopportune times.

The floor surface where we learn is vinyl tiling on concrete and although there is a partial, thin mat, I find the cold has exacerbated my problem. I suffer a lot with cold feet and although I wear socks to class, it doesn't help.

I would hate to give up dancing, yet obviously my feet are a necessary part of continuing!!! I am 45 and fairly healthy.'

Zaïda: Poor circulation can lead to cold hands and feet and muscle cramps.

I recommend you buy the book:

Hand Reflexology by Mildred Carter and Tammy Weber

PRENTICE HALL *http://www.phdirect.com*

In the meantime, try wearing thermal socks and soft shoes (like Jiffies) when you dance. Hope you can solve this problem.

WAITING 24 YEARS!

'I have wanted, for 24 years, to take belly dance lessons and I am going to try for the first time this next Monday. I am hoping we can modify some of the moves so I can do them and also hoping to lose some weight!'

Zaïda: :smile:: Welcome to the world of belly dance! ENJOY! you will find it helps enormously with a wide range of health issues. This is possibly the only exercise which works on the internal organs and not just arms, legs and heart/lungs as in aerobics etc.

Stimulating the internal organs helps your body to heal itself. You will also find that fat will turn to muscle; so do not watch those scales and feel you are not losing weight….muscle is heavier than fat. If you FEEL better, that is all that matters.

ENJOY! Have FUN!

BARING ALL IN THE STREETS OF LONDON

'I am an Australian living in the UK where we don't have the opportunity to belly dance, due to the weather. Do you have any hints or tips for me to keep warm whilst baring all in the streets of London?

I have always thought that belly dancing was a very fashionable and fantastic sport.

One day I will become a STAR!'

Zaïda: :smile:: If you look on my Dancing in Mackay page you will see a Link to Yasmin Asar, who teaches in London, UK.

Yasmin is a lovely person…she did a workshop here just over a year ago. SHE will keep you warm.

ADRENALIN

'I am 52 and have been bellydancing for 4 years and no-one believes I am over 35—especially when they see me in costume.

It's so true, what you say about the adrenalin high after dancing and being ready to party!

Keep the site going for us senior citizens…. '

Zaïda: :smile:: what you say about nobody believing your age when you dance…. is so true. I am told again and again that I look about 18 when I dance. Considering that I will be 65 on 31st July 2001, I can hardly believe this, but I get the comment repeatedly, so believe me…. I BELIEVE IT!

I have added a bit more to my Attitude page…you may like to take a look.

INSPIRED!

'Hi, Thought it would be nice to let you know that over the last three years dancing has become lots of fun just like you said it would.

First time I contacted you I was a beginner and doing child care. I kept up my dance classes and went to school to be an Administration Assistant…. all because you helped inspire me to reach for more at 50. Working as an Administration Assistant—and belly dancing, keeps me energized.'

Zaïda: I remember you well! I am so pleased you have grabbed life and done what YOU want.

HOW CAN YOU NOT DANCE?

'I loved your dance page. I have not danced in 5 years and after seeing your page, I am going to pull my costumes out of the closet and start using them again.'

Zaïda: How can you NOT dance? Dance wherever people will sit still long enough to watch…. dance for the people in the Nursing Homes…. they are the most appreciative audience you can find…. you will fill their day with SUNSHINE!

DANCE FOR SENIORS

'As a teacher of Dance for Seniors, I was disappointed not to be able to access the hyperlink for Dancing for Older Women.

My oldest students are 82'

Zaïda: It is so encouraging to hear of women of 82 still dancing.

Sometimes hyperlinks fail when the ISP is TOO BUSY.... which is happening more and more as people discover the WEB.

I hope you will try again....

CRIPPLING ILLNESS

'Hi Zaida! I don't know whether you're aware of it (maybe you are), but your web site is proving to be an inspiration for A LOT of older women! If you haven't already seen it, you may find the following web site interesting. It talks about how you helped someone heal from a crippling illness:

http://www.ladybarbara.net/bellyd.htm'

—**Shira**

Zaïda: I did not know this, but it gives me a truly warm, fuzzy feeling.

I have just spent 4 days at a convention for Older Women.... the Older Women's Network (OWN), where I conducted gentle exercise sessions, based on belly dance movements, each morning; a Workshop on Belly Dance on one of the days, then performed in the Variety Concert on the final night.

The ENERGY coming back to me from the audience of more than 70 Older Women was so INTENSE that I danced with more verve and excitement than I have ever danced before and had just about exhausted myself by the end of my 6 minute solo.

They were shouting and screaming for MORE! MORE! MORE! and I was thinking "I've HAD it!", but I gave them an encore...4 minutes, which I had ready. This encore is more of a 'fun' thing, than a serious display of belly dance.

I am still FLYING after this experience and then I get your email.. how HIGH can one fly? Thankyou so much...you have given me a HUGE lift. THANK YOU

—**Shira** 'Wow, your experience at that convention sounds INCREDIBLE! Many professional dancers go through an entire career without getting such intense response from an audience.

Which all goes to show there's more to performing than just running through a bunch of step combinations. You clearly felt a level of connection and respect for your audience even before you began to dance. They sensed it, which is why they responded to you the way they did.

Other dancers go on stage with their brains in the mode of "Look at me! I'm the star! Admire me!" I'm sure you had very different thoughts in your brain when you went on stage and that's what triggered the audience response.

The next time you feel tired or discouraged, you can think back to your high of this week and it'll lift your spirits. Isn't dance wonderful!'

COSTUME PATTERNS

'I am 46 this year and I would love to learn to bellydance. I love the costumes, but am not a small person.... I take a size 24dd bra and have enough difficulty finding attractive bras to wear everyday without attempting to find one suitable for bellydance. I do sew my own clothes and have looked for a pattern in the commercial books, but they don't size them in large sizes. Any suggestions would be great.'

Zaïda: There is absolutely no need for you to wear the cabaret costume of bra and skirt.... a full length dress with lots of layers of swirling chiffon would look fantastic.

EGYPTIAN CARTOUCHE

'I am a 47-year-old woman who discovered the art of belly dance in June 2000. I was "hooked" after my very first class and now take three classes a week! As a fuller-figured, middle-age woman with wide hips, a large "jelly-belly" and a very ample backside, I have found this dance form to be enlightening, refreshing, and one of the most freeing activities I have ever tried. When I'm dancing, I'm no longer just an older "fat" lady...I am a goddess, I am transformed, I am a divine desert diva!

There are enormous physical and emotional benefits that I have found through the dance. I am a breast cancer survivor and the dance has been restoring not only my physical strength, stamina and flexibility, but has helped restore my own sense of femininity and self-esteem, something the very nature of breast cancer tends to rob women of. Who knows...I may be the ONLY breast cancer surviving belly dancer!!

And you know what...my dance instructor, Morgiana, gave me the thrill of a lifetime in October 2000 when she asked me to join her performing dance troupe! Now I'm an apprentice in Egyptian Cartouche, based in Tempe, Arizona, and I perform several times a month in local restaurants within the Phoenix metropolitan area!

Your website was one of the very first I found when I started dancing and I thank you for helping give me the courage to keep going and not let my self-imposed feelings about my body stop me. Now I'm not just a woman...I am a dancer...I am an artist.'

MEDIEVAL FAIR

'I too am a 47 year old breast cancer survivor and have been taking lessons for about six months now.

I know what she (Egyptian Cartouche) is talking about when your woman-hood is taken away.

I have been having so much fun and I feel graceful and sexy again. I am performing with the troupe in one week at our local Medieval Fair.'

INSTRUCTIONAL VIDEOS

'I am a belly dancer who has not been dancing for a few years and wishes to get back into it. I am looking for a "how to" video and was hoping that you could supply me with info on where to obtain it.

Where I live in Washington there is nothing of the sort as you can imagine. I am finding all kinds of websites for bellydance performances but no instructional.'

Zaïda: I suggest you go to my Links page and click on The Art of Middle Eastern Dance. This is **Shira's** site and I am sure you will find instructional videos there...

I would recommend Yasmin Asar's video, (see my Dancing In Mackay page) but she only produces it in PAL, which won't play in the USA unless you have a multi-format VCR.

STAR DANCER with ISIS

'I found your site from the link on **Ankh's** page; I too am a student of Isis, and recently had the honour of being named as one of the Star Dancers.

Although I am only 30, I just wanted to let you know that I found your site to be wonderful!!!

The advice that you give is so true to belly dancers of all ages. I would like to comment on the Repartee question (I think from 1999) in which the husband questioned you on his wife's 'jelly belly'. I have a 'jelly belly' also, and I recently decided not to show my belly when I dance. This decision came because I felt I needed to concentrate more on the dance itself than on what people are thinking of me and whether or not they are trying to count my stretch marks.'

Zaïda: PLEASE! say 'hello' to Ankh for me when next you see him. I have found his support so valuable, particularly when I first set up my web page and he was so encouraging. I was THRILLED!!

I am beginning to feel in agreement with your sentiments that you prefer not to display your belly—in order to let people concentrate on the dance and not the belly. I think my next costume will be a good deal more discreet.

CAESAREAN

'I LOVE and appreciate your website! I am 30 lbs overweight, 47 yr old, 5' at most. I don't like exercise because of my over-weightiness in the belly (from a C-section childbirth) and hips.

I love to dance but have lost the rock 'n roll moves. I decided to try belly dancing. The name implies it would get right to the needed area.

There is no one in this area to teach or show me, so I bought a belly-dancing exercise tape, "The Goddess Workout", by Dolphina. She shows the Camel, Snake and hip rotations with a good warm-up and cool-down; but it is obvious to me (or so it looks) that she has never had children. That's why I was uplifted and enjoyed you so much! I fit right in!

Because of my C-Section, my lower belly is what I most need to workout. What exercises or routines of bellydance would most firm up this area?

For your courage and determination I want to congratulate you.... although your figure and energy level are all the congratulations you need I am sure!'

Zaïda: Welcome to the world of belly dance. Firstly, I gave birth to a boy, then a girl, then had an hysterectomy at the age of 32. I think this would be a very similar operation to a Caesarean, except there is no further risk of pregnancy.

I have VERY wide hips—childbearing hips—from my Austrian/Dutch maternal forebears; but that is my skeleton and no amount of slimming will diminish this....

Bellydancing will control your weight and fine up your body whilst you are enjoying yourself.

About weight-loss.... the body is like a car engine and needs fuel to run. Unfortunately, unlike a car engine, if you put in too much fuel, it will not just overflow and run out onto the ground, it will congeal into fat.

Ignore your early training about eating all the food on your plate. The person who put the food on your plate has no idea how hungry you are. When you feel you have had enough STOP EATING. Bin the rest....

Also, a Diuretic is helpful to rid your body of excess fluids....amazing how fat they can make you look.

I urge you to see a dietician, as you could have a food allergy and this causes the body to store fluid in order to protect itself.

OR, you may be on the wrong form of HRT and need to change brands...makes a difference.

Once your body tones up and you develop your muscles, you may find your weight does not drop below a certain point.... muscle is much heavier than fat. If you look and feel good...IGNORE the scales.

Set yourself up with a 'routine' and do this EVERY day. A warm-up, some belly dance moves and a cool-down. As you learn more moves and your fitness increases, your routine will get longer and more energetic. You will soon find you cannot do without this heart-starter in the mornings, and will feel stiff and dull unless you do your 'routine' every day. Don't feel despondent if you cannot do a move you have seen, just keep trying and suddenly it will be there.

VERY INTERESTED

'Hi! I am very interested in your page on belly dancing for older women, and I was wondering if you could email me some more information on this topic?'

Zaïda: I have put practically all I know about belly dancing on my website, but if you care to go to the Links page, **Shira's** site 'The Art of Middle Eastern Dance' is very extensive and informative. Also the Danish site, which you can access through the Aladdin's lamp on my Dancing page, is very good as **Botticelli** has put up little videos of the basic moves.

If you are in the U.K. you may like to look at my 'In Mackay page', at the very bottom is a Link to **Yasmin Asar** who teaches in London and she is a LOVELY person. She came to Oz last year and has put out a beginners/intermediate video on PAL format.

If you are an older woman who is a bit shy about joining a local class.... DON'T BE!

Belly dancers (the type of women who are attracted to this form of dance) are all lovely people and will be very welcoming and helpful. If you are shy about your body, take a look at **Seleka** *www.bellydanceny.com/seleka.html*

Zaïda

0-595-20948-3

Printed in the United States
38335LVS00006B/397-402